About the Author

After obtaining his degree in medicine, M B B S, and working for three years in a rural community in Kerala, India, Kottiyattil K Aravind came to England in 1965. While he was working as a Plastic Surgeon in Edinburgh he became a Fellow of the Royal College of Surgeons of Edinburgh. In 1975 he had to abandon the hospital career for family reasons and became a GP in a small town-practice in northern England. He took serious interest in the use of medical hypnosis to enlighten himself while working in a routine general practice, at the same time benefitting his patients. He served the British Society of Medical and Dental Hypnosis as Hon. Secretary. As a strong academic, he was convinced about the high value of the use and the benefit of hypnosis in medicine, which motivated him to create the postgraduate "Diploma and Masters Courses in Medical Hypnosis" based in the Medical Faculty of the University of Sheffield. Working with colleagues it became a reality in 1989. At that time it was the first of its kind in the world. To his further achievement in the field of Medical Hypnosis, he co-authored with Dr Michael Heap, the Fourth Edition of Hartland's Medical and Dental Hypnosis, Churchill Livingston (Harcourt International) 2002, ISBN 0-443-07217-5. Since his retirement from general practice, struggling through his lifelong disability of dyslexia and narcolepsy, KKA managed to publish his book about the "Question and Answer Model©™" which in his experience is the most effective method of treatment to **set free** millions of bereaved around the world from the suffering of harmful grief. He strongly believes that it can create a world with peace and love based on understanding, a world free of hatred and destruction.

Grief – How It Harms and How To Cure It

A REVOLUTIONARY SINGLE SESSION APPROACH TO ACHIEVE
A COMPLETE RELEASE FROM THE SUFFERING CAUSED BY ANY
FORM OF GRIEF OF ANY ORIGIN AND ANY DURATION AND TO
REGAIN NORMALITY FOR THE REST OF LIFE

IT CAN BE DONE ONLY THROUGH A TOTALLY DIFFERENT
UNDERSTANDING OF HOW GRIEF GENERATES HARM IN THE
BEREAVED, WHICH IS DESCRIBED

BY

THE QUESTION AND ANSWER MODEL©™

Dr Kottiyattil K Aravind

First Edition

Published in 2016

Copy wright-2016 of all contents to Dr Kottiyattil K Aravind

doctoraravind@sky.com United Kingdom

ISBN: 1530479169

ISBN 13: 9781530479160

Dedicated to my wife Carol

Contents

Introduction

"Question and Answer Model©™" is an original creation by Dr Kottiyattil K Aravind (KKA). He had worked on the model for over twenty years. It had evolved through a lengthy, bit-by-bit process, involving logical questioning and thinking through sensible answers. Every step of the development of his revolutionary treatment programme was discussed giving free and equal input from the bereaved persons whom he had treated for 'harmful grief'. The term 'harmful grief' is used by KKA in his classification of grief, which will be explained in detail later. In his understanding, grief is an inevitable emotional state a bereaved would experience, which often wain as the life carries on and that is just as another inevitable process. In some bereaved, they have to endure the harm for the rest of their lifetime or at least for an unpredictable part of their life. During the process of his in-depth analysis in the search for a cure to the harm caused by that emotional aberrant, called grief, he had to abandon hitherto existing theories and approaches for treating grief in order to develop a totally fresh but different approach in helping the bereaved.

Mainly because the hitherto therapies involving measures, sometimes simple or very complicated, taken by both common people and academic experts alike, had failed to remove the harmful effect completely and permanently, KKA set his search upon a completely different pathway to understand the dynamics of how grief causes harm not to all the bereaved, but only in some of them, even though to a considerable number, while many of the grief stricken do not endure any harm at all. Current available approaches help sufferers of grief to cope by accommodating the harm as part of a slightly better normality in their life. The harm may be manifested as both physical and mental/behavioural dysfunction, albeit with a lesser force in some victims those who had the benefit of traditional therapy, while others just carried on with fully fledged dysfunctions right up to their own death.

The failure of presently available approaches in making the grief a totally harmless process is because, up until now, the suggested dynamics of how it harms have also failed to be robustly convincing. The success of the solutions, which would be automatically robust, if only the understanding of the dynamics could be applied equally to all harmful grief. KKA was looking for a treatment package involving just one or two sessions, as that was all he could afford in his general practice timetable. More than to overcome the time and economical restraints, he wanted to set free the victims within the fastest timescale, because of the terrible suffering they had to endure from the harmful grief. The suffering vary enormously and often untold, not only between the bereaved, but also within the people around them, who are made to suffer as well, because of the dysfunctional behaviour of the bereaved. One of the inevitable components of harmful grief is the negative judgement, such as guilt, hatred, anger, shame and hurt, either towards themselves or towards others. The negative emotions may be of extreme intensity and may turn the aggrieved to commit terrible tragedies of revenge, murders, destructions and occasionally all out wars. Self-guilt and self-hatred are more common, which may lead to self-punishment because of the denial of their worthiness or the underplaying of their abilities creating the feeling of uselessness. Worst of all and more often, according to KKA, is the germination of many forms of illnesses. Paradoxically there were a few good things that had come out of harmful grief in human history, as the bereaved went about compensating their emotions by becoming overgenerous to the world at large, for example the building of Taj Mahal and many monuments like that, as well as founding numerous charitable organisations. The most famous of them all was what King Asoka did in India, the popularisation of Buddhism.

KKA wanted not only an instant change over from harming grief to a positive normality prevailed with love, joy and happiness giving the bereaved a productive functional life for their future, but also such turn-around has to be none less than an absolute cure and stay cured for the rest of their life. He knew the task was a tall order, but worked relentlessly over a period of ten years, until he managed to create the **"Question and Answer Model ©™"**. Even though it was impossible to conduct a controlled study within the constraints of his small town general practice he had used the model in numerous of his own patients and friends, who were suffering from harmful grief of duration as recent as a few days up to as old as thirty years duration. He had used the model in children as young as ten years and adults as old as eighty years. The model was found effective also in the prevention of harmful grief in prospective bereaved who would be expecting impending death of a loved one. At the same time, it had helped people, who were expecting to die soon from non-treatable illnesses to become more positive and productive during their last part of the journey, and so benefiting all the people involved. One of the bereaved, who had received such help from KKA, commented soon after the death of her husband that, "I am not angry that he died". During his work in the dermatology department in the local district hospital and to the surprise of many, some of the 'intractable skin conditions' were cured, following the treatment of the underlying grief using his model. From the personal feedback by the patients a great number of them have achieved remarkable resolution and regained normality in their life. Because of the success, which he was getting time after time, case after case; he had given workshops in the Hypnosis Society and had taught the students of Diploma and Masters Courses in Hypnosis in Sheffield University. His colleagues and students entreated him to publish this work.

Struggling with his life long disability of dyslexia and narcolepsy it took him twenty years to publish this book about the "Question and Answer Model©™". He has taken every effort to make the contents of this book easily understood by people of all walks of life, professionals as well as ordinary individuals. He genuinely hopes that many therapists of many disciplines will apply his "Question and Answer Model©™" in their effort to help their patients suffering from "harmful grief". He, KKA is looking forward to a contribution however small towards creating a world with peace and love based on understanding, a world free of hatred and destruction.

Acknowledgement

KKA likes to extend his heart-felt gratitude to the students who had encouraged him to publish this book and above all to the bereaved, who have immensely contributed in the development the model as well as benefitted from the treatment received from KKA. The many benefactors of the treatment offered by KKA had explicitly paid tributes to the model itself and that was the driving force in KKA to accomplish this work, which took well over twenty years to do.

KKA wishes to express special gratitude to his wife Carol to whom the book is dedicated for her invaluable help and encouragement in the creation of this book.

Chapter One

Grief A Revolutionary, "Question and Answer Model©™" and Single Session Treatment

This model is developed and practiced with great success By Kottiyattil K Aravind (KKA)

"Where there is love the life is full
No life is a single piece
One fragment upon another, upon another, makes one life
So there should be equally different fragments of love to fill one life.
The perfect love is like the perfect pearl on a beach;
Without which the beach is nothing.
That pearl makes any life more than a matter of living."

(Philosophy of Life and Love by Aravind)

Definition of grief by KKA - *Grief is the emotional aberration, sequel to the loss by death or separation perceived as permanent as death, of a loved person, animal or an object of sentiment constituting a new behavioural mould within which the bereaved is constrained.*

The word *'grief'* was derived from *gravare*, version of the Latin word *gravis*, meaning heavy, to denote deep sorrow or intense mourning. The word *'bereaved'* came from German *be-reafian,* meaning to be robbed or forcibly deprived of anything valued. The grieving persons are the bereaved.

Grief is a spontaneous 'no-option response' in the bereaved, initiated simultaneously with the realisation of the loss. Grief may manifest as simply experiencing sorrow or sadness. On the other hand it may be associated with dysfunctional psychosocial behaviours, such as extreme hatred, revenge, murder, feuds and wars and conversely guilt, sacrifice and extreme generosity. The mental health changes vary between anxiety, sexual malfunction, inability to contemplate any aspect of happiness, performance deprivation, difficult inter personal relationship, depression, agoraphobia, mental paralysis, schizoid state and even suicide. Somatization may present as simple as skin eczema and headache to almost any illness, even cancer due to possible immunosuppression.

Historical orientation of grief

Literally thousands of books are published connected with grief. Many of them are based on personal experience like C.S. Lewis - 'A Grief Observed', Barbara Want - 'A Story of Love and Loss'. There are plenty of novels, poems, plays and films with grief at their heart, e.g. "Gideon's Daughter", "The man who was Peter Pan", "Bogus", "The memory of Water" and so on. Unlimited analytical and research papers exists in the literature by authors skilled in counselling, psychology or psychiatry from Freud, Elizabeth Kubler-Ross, Parks, Strobes, Lieberman to Worden.

One of the tragedies of earlier medical education and the health care system is that the hospital based medical practice is heavily orientated on specific diagnosis and prescribed treatments. Historically, with hands on heart, many medical professionals as well as the public at large would admit that they are reluctant to talk out loud about the philosophy of death and its affect, mainly grief. Most of us would choose rather to shy away and avoid entering into any constructive conversation about grief. Instead most us leave the subject to the very few of those who specialise in it. This apathy spontaneously creates indifference towards the subject of grief. Whether that apathy is a shield to the fear of exposing oneself and being unable to cope with the upsurge of personal feelings within, or it might be merely a matter of ignorance. For whatever reasons, such indifference would inevitably make one overlook the most devastating affects of grief as the fundamental causative agent in both dysfunctional behaviour and physical diseases in the millions of bereaved.

KKA had observed during his ten-year (1965-1975) hospital service in the UK that, there might be an unintentional tendency to dismiss failures in the prescribed treatments, either as patient's non-compliance, or patients wanting to be sick for secondary gains. Regretfully, the failed cases may finally be discharged as hysteria or malingering. Apart from a very few people feigning sickness the great majority of the illnesses are genuine. Because the 'harmful grief' has remained as an integral part of their everyday life for a long time, the patients themselves did not expect grief could be the cause of their illness. So also the medical professionals fall into the same trap. The end result was that the patients failed to respond to all conventional treatments. Over the years (1975 -2004), working in general practice and running hypnosis clinics for intractable cases in the dermatology department in the local general hospital, KKA had exposed the underlying grief in many cases as the root cause of the resistance to conventional treatments. Treatment of the grief had not only alleviated their presenting illnesses, but also changed their life for better. It is not difficult to underpin the roll of grief in many cases. It only requires thinking of the possibility of grief having a part in the dynamics of many intractable physical, emotional and functional disorders and explaining to the patients that it may have some influence in the non-response to treatment and even the origin of their problem. If that is the case curing the harmful grief completely will have a high chance of curing the illness as well. It is time every one involved in health care to be aware of the possibility of grief as one of the causes of the presenting problem, especially when the textbook interventions are failing. *Patients almost never volunteer to mention grief, unless specifically asked for. With the exception of a few specialists in dealing with grief, almost all people believe that to have grief and to endure the affects of grief are looked upon as not only normal, but also inevitably the right thing to have. Therefore their approach to their presenting illness with absolute conviction that the cause of their illness is separate from the grief they are carrying.* The unawareness of grief might be the cause of many illnesses amongst the caring professionals, the issue of grief will remain irrelevant as a matter of fact in the management of diseases, whether mental, physical or both. Any tendency amongst medical doctors and dentists to put grief as a peripheral trivia would be to the peril of the patients.

Educational establishments also need to be trained to explore the possibility of hidden grief amongst children in education, when they exhibit misbehaviour out of their previous good character or show unexplained changes in their performance or struggling to hold attention. In the same way changes in parental attitudes towards their own children or even to the educational staff might point towards underlying grief. It might be as simple as that they are grieving the loss of their pet animal, for example, one case treated by KKA for school phobia associated with excessive vomiting while in school was due to grief from the loss of his pet dog.

Normal and Abnormal grief and the available therapies

It is beyond the scope of this mini book to get into the detailed exploration of symptomatology, innumerable theories and interventions, as there is an ocean of them in the literature.   KKA recommends, for interested parties to read, "Handbook of Bereavement, Theory, research and intervention" Ed. By M. S. Strobe, W. Strobe and R. O. Hansson (1993/2006).

Therefore only a brief overview of the historical background is given below.

Normal grief

Suggested stages of normal grief are initially shock, denial, numbness and disbelief, changing into anger, compromise and acceptance, leading to depression; progressing through a period of mourning, expressing emotional, physical and social sufferings and a period of emotional reckoning, and eventually the re-establishment of the world of normality. Such a course of grieving or mourning is often quoted as "normal grief".

Abnormal Grief

Grief that falls outside the normal has many adjectives, for example – pathological, abnormal, absent, hidden, unresolved, atypical, morbid, neurotic, intensified and prolonged, disabling, chronic, inhibited, delayed, dysfunctional, truncated, distorted, complicated, somatised grief and so on.

Grief had been categorised based on its associated symptoms permutated with multidimensional factors related to the deceased such as the social status, gender and age of the dead and type and circumstances of death, as well as implied with the bereaved in their future relationships, availability of support opportunities, the varied path of recovery and readjustments and so forth. To name a few of the symptoms, they would be shock, numbness, emotional pain, conflict of love, pain of loss of love, loneliness, feeling incomplete, crying, anger, guilt, anxiety, fear, helplessness, apathy, relief, regrets, acceptance or disbelief, altered perception, indulgence, altered faith, depression, habit disorders, post traumatic stress disorder, somatic symptoms, personality disorders, physiological, immunological, neuro-endocrinological, psychoneuroimmunalogical and so on.

Historically, therapy stretches only to help the bereaved to cope with the pain and the problems. Some of the professional therapists utilise the models of psychoanalysis and its variant psychodynamics. A few of the strategies are self adjustments, involvement of friends and kin, religious guidance, self help groups, supports in finance and services, profession-al counselling, Cruse counselling, Freudian psychotherapy, attachment psychotherapy, psychodynamic crisis intervention, dynamic psychother-apy, behavioural therapies, cognitive therapies, cognitive-behavioural therapies, bereavement counselling exploring important issues related to the bereaved person such as relationship, the loss, social support, other stressors, background, achieving goals and family variables, traditional psychiatric-mental health interventions and pharmacological intervention mostly antidepressants and tranquilisers.

Most bereaved people will make progress in some way or other, but stop short of a complete cure of the hurt in the carriage of grieving. All the bereaved, whether they had previous therapies or not, attending KKA for further help had expressed that they always carried a feeling of in-completeness since the loss of their loved-one. They never were able to get rid of the negative attitudes associated with their grief, such as anger, hate, guilt etc. Metaphorically speaking, they have lost one half of their emotional person along with the loss of their loved-one and so they continued to live with the remaining half only. Many cases remain non-re-sponsive to historical therapies and might even get worse because of the repetitions of the hurting process while undergoing those interventions. The very interventions invariably involve repetitions and re-emphasises of the underlying cause of the 'harmful grief', which will be described later. The above group of therapies and help either imposes restricted time scale not uncommonly ending the therapy half way to the need of the bereaved, or they can be very prolonged and expensive. In other words, apart from the new model evolved by KKA, in his knowledge, rarely any of the currently practiced therapies can deliver either a *complete cure* or a total turn around the life of the bereaved to normality. Literarily, at the finish of KKA's one-session treatment, the bereaved can feel 'complete' or 'wholesome' in themselves enabling them to regain their full functional potential. If they choose to, it would even enable them to have fresh love-relationships without reservations.

BRIEF ACCOUNTS OF SOME OF THE HISTORICAL MODELS

a). John Bowlby (Bowlby, 1961) describes acute grief as a frustrated form of search for the lost one and equates the pain of loss to the pain of separation or abandonment based on his work with attachment theory. In the experience of the author none of the patients of had ever indicated that any such notion had ever passed through their mind. Activities such as going to the grave side, keeping memorabilia, behaving as if the person had not died, led many to say that the bereaved was in denial or not accepting the truth of the loss. However during the in depth discussions between KKA and the bereaved, another explanation had been revealed for the above mentioned behaviour. They were searching for answers to the many questions, which were recurrently troubling their mind; and such questions had intimate connections with those memorabilia and/or the deceased persons themselves.

b). Thomas D Eliot in the 1930s ("The Adjustive Behaviour of Bereaved Families, *Social Forces, VIII (1930) 546,* as quoted in the book of "The Dynamic of Grief", *David K Switzer,* Abingdon Press, New York, 1970, page 22) had attempted to place grief within psychological parameters as the resurgence of trauma, frustration and forced abandonment of habits or wishes following the death of a loved one.

Living with a loved-one cultivates in a person the habit of demands and dependency on that loved person. Such rooted activities or memories could become a kind of stimulant essential for the person, in this case the bereaved, to function smoothly. When the loved-one has gone, these associated habits and needs are no longer available to stimulate normality, while the memories of them remain alive in the mind of the bereaved. Severe frustration develops and probably manifests as harmful grief. The bereaved may feel helpless and powerless, may even feel loss of identity, which leads to fear and anxiety. It may be so, that the intensity of harmful grief is proportionate to the prior intensity of love and dependency. If that is the dynamics, it would demand the bond of dependency along with associated memories are to be broken, in order to remove the harming affect of grief and that is extremely difficult. The realisation of KKA is in fact the opposite.   Such memories are to be strengthened and not to be weakened, because all the bereaved have uniquely insisted that they do not want to forget or forgo any of such memories whether they were good memories or bad memories. In fact the bereaved would go further to say that the more they think about the missing help and guidance, it had the effect of making them realise that it would be up to them to swim or sink and so wanting to be more self-reliant to cope with their life in future. In the model, which KKA has developed, the bereaved will be told at the start of the therapy that they will not be required to forget anything; on the contrary they will have the opposite benefit of "they will never have to feel that are missing the loved one, metaphorically they will be with them all the time by virtue of the constant awareness of the wisdom that had been passed on by the deceased". Case history No.14 illustrate the issue.

*The dynamics of how grief can produce mental and physical harm in the bereaved as well as making the bereaved to harm others are **entirely due** to the existence of negative emotions of guilt, anger and hatred attached with unanswered questions arising from the circumstances surrounding the death. This new understanding, which is fundamentally different from all the other forms of therapies, makes the foundation of KKA's therapeutic modal, which has proved most successful in the treatment of harmful grief.*

c). The psychoanalytical domain may underpin all adult anxiety or mourning as the replication or recalled experience of the separation anxiety of the child from the mother, often called "infantile mourning". The suffering in grief is the adult anxiety having the same characteristics. Freud would say all anxiety starts from the early experience of separation of the mother, compounded with Oedipus hostility and guilt.

The anxiety and fear response is not a new invention in grief. They are the same reactions or responses, which since the time of birth, an individual gets accustomed to or conditioned in situations of trauma of any kind, not necessarily separation. We learn the experience of 'fear' from possible danger. This is a natural and essential instinct for the survival and preservation of the species. Fear response is generated when one is left alone and exposed to predators and not being guarded safely. The process of the experience of 'anxiety' is secondary to the experience of fear, which is generated when there is a perceived threat to the existence of the self. Anxiety is a warning signal, making the organism prepared and ready to spring into action on future occasions of threat, equipped with various physiological alterations in the physical system. These temporary changes in the body and mind are perceived at an emotional level as pain, sometimes as physical pain, along with other manifestations of anxiety.

Assumptions may be made in the psychoanalytical world the grief will be expressed in its entirety in other forms of suffering in those bereaved who failed to express fully, all the so-called manifests of grief. This indicates that in helping with grief one should strive to make the bereaved travel through the full course of grief, whatever the full course may be, and failure to do so will allow the suffering from grief to continue, while the need to mourn will persist and may manifest itself in other forms of illness such as depression and so on.

In the experience of KKA, while treating many bereaved with grief of all kinds, he has come across no absolute measurable unites of grief either quantitatively or qualitatively nor has a road map with defined boundary lines, which can be applied in all the cases of bereaved. KKA believes that grief is very subjective and so stands different in each case. It also means the manifestations are unique to one bereaved from the other and it may include physical or mental suffering which may start from the very moment of the death.

Psychoanalytical model of Denial, searching, Yearning

Often writers and speakers conducting workshops about grief mention that some bereaved switch into a state of denial, in other words the bereaved does not want to accept or admit that their loved one has indeed died. They do things as if the dead person is still alive, like cooking for him/her, placing dinner plates where he/she usually sit for dinner, leaving everything to stand still like in the story of Sleeping Beauty. As long as the bereaved continue to grieve, they may create a shrine in their home. They may place perishable things like their favourite food or toys and gadgets etc. near their graveside or in the shrine in the house. In the opinion of KKA such comments are overzealous remarks. The analysis of some writers go to the extent of saying that when the bereaved go to the grave more often and talking to the dead person at grave side or similar behaviour are signs of attempting to make contact with their loved ones, as they are in denial of the death of the loved one. In the experience of KKA treating many people for harmful grief, no one had ever mentioned that they were in denial; meaning neither they did think that the person has not died nor they were trying to pretend nothing had happened. On deeper discussion they all said that such a notion had never crossed their thoughts. In fact, what KKA believes that they were searching for answers to the many questions, which were recurrently troubling their mind; and such questions had intimate connections with those memorabilia and/or the deceased persons themselves

The only advice that KKA would give to the bereaved is not to take any advice from anybody including KKA regarding how, when and what the bereaved should or would feel, do or behave from the time when the death has occurred to any time in their life. Every individual is different in many ways of how their life needs to be and there are equally different ways to get it.

d) Analysts had identified four stages of grief as far back as 1940s. Grief passes through from an immediate stage expressed with shock and wailing lasting up to several hours following the death, through a second stage of being detached, a third stage of transition and the final stage of getting back to active life. Several people have propounded the idea of grief being a staged process. One of the foremost of these has been Elizabeth Kubler-Ross. She had defined grief in 5 stages in her book - "On Grief and Grieving".

KKA had observed that the idea of staging grief unfortunately can be taken too literally and applied too rigidly. People do not always exhibit all the so-called stages and may move from one to another and back again at various times rather than in an orderly progression.

Chapter Two

Grief – A Revolutionary "Question and Answer Model"©™ and Single Session Treatment

The Question and Answer model can be understood from the following 4 sections

1. Evolution of the Question and Answer (Q & A) model.
2. Formation of Question & Answer model and how it explains the dynamics of grief.
3. Harmless grief and Harmful grief
4. Treatment of grief using Q & A model, for a complete resolution, all in a single session.

Evolution of the Question & Answer Model – Q & A Model

Amongst his UK practice population, in spite of its comparative wealth and privileges, KKA was taken aback with the presentation of sudden and severe swings of the mental and physical health as an aftermath of bereavement. The levels of such changes may vary from mild to extreme of negative feelings like **guilt, anger, hurt, hatred, shame and unworthiness**. Growing up and working as a medical practitioner in the rural communities of Kerala, South India, KKA recognised a stark contrast in the high level of harmful grief in the UK society against the remarkable lack of harmful grief in his native community.

Death is universal and no one can escape from it. So also everyone will have to go through grief sometime in his or her lifetime.

In 1975 KKA entered into general practice in a northern township in the UK. Soon he became aware of the devastating effect of grief amongst his patients. It became one of his major quests to find a robust therapeutic process to help them. He earnestly wanted to help those people. The search began. Soon he realised that he needed to understand the innermost core of the reasons for the disparity between Keralians and his UK patients. He built the foundations of his quest by giving unlimited time, hundreds of hours outside his basic time of duty, in conversation with the bereaved. Because of his absolutely non-judgmental attitude and ever-present empathy during such unconditional enquiries, the bereaved felt free to open up and express their very intimate feelings generated by the loss of their loved ones. They revealed not only their negative emotions, but also certain special thoughts that *'pass through their mind, relentlessly, during most of their waking hours'*.

Almost nine out of ten bereaved people, who had opened up and expressed such thoughts, did it for the first time since the loss of their loved ones. They told KKA he was the first person they were able to speak about the true reasons, as they perceived based on their own judgments, which created the negative feelings. In their own statements, they would not have ever mentioned those thoughts to any other souls, including their beloveds and most trusted friends. The reason for the secrecy was that their negative feelings were attached to very special personal thoughts. In their judgment, those thoughts were loaded with guilt and so they were deeply ashamed as well as afraid of the reactions, which might follow by exposing that side of themselves to the outside world. They also believed that by telling someone however trusted they might be, it would not help to make any change in those thoughts. More powerfully they entrenched themselves in the belief that they should not allow anyone to change them, because those thoughts equated with love, justice and fairness between them and the dead person. Therefore they had to hold on to them at any cost and could not allow anything or anybody attempting to change it. KKA believes that social and family constructs are practical issues, which the bereaved have to deal with for the re-organisation of future, but not necessarily they generate harmful grief.

Formation of the Question & Answer Model and how it explains the dynamics of grief.

KKA decided to build the model to understand how grief germinates in the psyche of the bereaved and how it can turn in some cases to harm the very bereaved persons and persons associated with them by virtue of the suffering of the bereaved. Such an in depth knowledge is essential if the harming has to be removed fully and permanently in every case. KKA decided to choose materials obtained by listening wholesomely to what the bereaved had to say, meaning *"what goes through their thoughts as the whole truth"* to be used as the only building blocks for his model. More than that, he believed that any attempt to interpret or to manipulate what they had to say in order to fit into the traditional pre-existing models, would distort the naked truths. One fact that stared in his face was that within his knowledge, all the ancient and modern models of grief therapy had never achieved a complete cure, meaning a full turn around in their life to normality and also to enable them to remember or talk about the dead person with ease and little pain. KKA wanted an entirely new concept of how grief might harm and so a completely new model to treat it without the slightest intrusion of the existing ideas and models of grief therapy, which he believed might corrupt his model and might repeat the failures of the past. KKA believes that harmful grief is purely an emotional and very private affair to the bereaved, because it is constructed solely by the bereaved, *quite consciously*, through internal self-dialogue.

When some one dies in Kerala, the mourners would exhibit their raw emotions by crying their heart out. There are no norms for expressing one's sorrow and everyone respects and allows others to express freely without fear of causing offence. What more unique an occasion to do so? The core characteristic of that kind of mourning is that, individuals will cry out loudly, all their good and wrong doings, which had happened in *their lifetime,* and it may concern the deceased also. The wailing is not only perfectly acceptable, but also is encouraged, asking forgiveness from the dead, as well as forgiving the dead for all their mistakes.

Hardly any secrets will be left after the first day of the mourning, including the secrets related to the dead as well. All the wailing dialogue is in the **format of questions and answers**. If anyone did not get the answers, as it is not possible especially from the dead, someone else in the wailing group would speak on behalf of the dead, as the mourners will be sitting around the dead person, to make every item of the outpourings all-inclusive. Such a catharsis helps to prevent the manufacture of guilt, anger or hatred. More importantly, it will be a full family affair. Children of all ages are routinely included, which gives the perfect opportunity for everyone to grow accustomed to a healthy way to react to the loss. The funeral itself and the rituals immediately afterwards are heavily weighted with gestures of goodbyes to the departed. A few days later there will be a feast to celebrate the life of the loved one, underpinning the end of mourning and time to get back to normality. Thereafter people will feel free to talk about the bygone events and memories inclusive of those matters associated with the dead. They will talk about the deceased as if that the person is alive, and the conversations will include both good and bad about the deceased making the memory, a uniquely complete one.

KKA noticed an important difference between the UK patients and the Keralian community. The UK patients ask the same number of similar questions, but they do it mostly in secret within their own mind, while holding quite steadfast to the 'stiff upper lip persona' outwardly. They admit that they rarely would have dared to whisper their questions to any body, until and most often for the first time to KKA during the session of grief therapy in the congenial environment of trust and friendship, which KKA creates during his sessions. When KKA gave them fully satisfying answers to such questions, often using metaphors (*as KKA understand, a metaphor is something which is familiar to the listener, is used as a tool to explain something which is difficult to understand or to accept as an explanation*) the bereaved would invariably make remarks like, 'that has taken a load off my mind', 'why didn't I think of that', 'is it true', 'I am so relieved to hear it'. They spontaneously initiate the process of returning to the long awaited normality of their life.

The author took the decision in the 1980s to look at how the human mind works when grief strikes, based on the above observations which he was making, not only in the context of grief but also in other challenging or unpleasant situations. For a while he kept himself out of using any psycho-analytical or intricate formulae to explain his own evolving model, which he wanted to keep highly flexible as a fluid idea with no boundaries. Day after day the sufferers knew exactly what was going through their thoughts and feelings. They were capable of narrating the whole problem. He believed that there were neither hidden things in the unconscious that they had no comprehension of, nor there was any mysticism about it.

Faced with a tragic event, whether it is little or great, and death being the greatest, all human beings, without exception as creatures of reason-ing, will analyse from all angles of that event. They would want to know if there was anything at all, which might be different from what actually had happened; or anything at all would or could have prevented that tragedy altogether or at least delayed the final departure in the cases of the termi-nally ill. There is only one methodology to make such analysis by anyone and that is by asking a lot of *questions*. Questions about the illness, how it was treated, was the roll of everyone involved with the deceased con-ducted correctly and was it appropriately timed, were there any mistakes, who made the mistakes if any, was there enough compassion and so on and on. Every *question* demands *answers.* KKA believes such ques-tioning is purely for a matter of survival, and is essential for the preserva-tion of the human species. It is an automatic and natural reaction to any catastrophe, especially in grief.

He formulated the Question and Answer Model around 1994. He was working full time in general practice, at the same time heavily involved with the courses of Diploma and Masters in Clinical Hypnosis at Sheffield University. KKA was one of the founders of those courses. He took the opportunity to share the idea with the experienced professionals from all disciplines of medicine, dentistry and psychology, which helped him to consolidate the model. The postgraduate students, highly qualified professional in their fields, enthusiastically accepted the model. KKA was invited to give workshops to the members of British Society of Medical and Dental Hypnosis, demonstrating how it worked with real cases. All such workshops proved the validity of the model and the outpour of enthusiasms amongst the students encouraged him to publish the idea. At the same time KKA have treated many cases within his practice population, local cancer support group and Dermatology Department in the local General Hospital, with a high degree of success with one-session treatment, which convinced KKA himself of the credibility and the unparalleled benefit in treating harmful grief, using his model of 'Question and Answers'.

HARMLESS GRIEF AND HARMFUL GRIEF

KKA likes to classify grief or even to describe it, only on the basis whether the *bereaved is in need of treatment or not. Therefore KKA classifies grief into 'harmless grief' when the bereaved is getting on with life as normal as can be and not afflicted psycho-somatically; and 'harmful grief' when the bereaved requires help or treatment for mental and/or somatic dysfunction.*

HARMLESS GRIEF

It is generally accepted that a good number of the bereaved will get through the inevitable sadness from the loss of their loved ones, without any substantial altercations with their normal life. The bereaved may feel sadness for many years and all it demands is an occasional weep at a convenient time and place, either on their own or in the company of trusted persons. As long as it does not affect the near normality in their life, the *grief is harmless.* All bereaved ask questions. A few of them will produce answers using their intelligence and lifetime learning. Some of them might get answers by listening to other people. Whatever sources the answers may come from, as long as they are able to accept and integrate the answers with their belief system, the bereaved will be contented in their life because they know that the best possible has been done for the deceased. Therefore the grief will remain as a harmless one and that group of bereaved does not require any treatment. It is only right for them to be left alone.

HARMFUL GRIEF

The story is different in many others, who also ask similar questions. Burdened with the greatest tragedy of their life, the loss of a loved one, most of the questions are likely to be irrational. Some of them can be based on ill-understood medical details. Some questions are about misconduct from professionals and other people involved in the care of the deceased. Yet again, the emotional agony often construes the perception about the deeds of those people and for that matter their own deeds. In the context of grief, reality is not allowed to prevail. Instead the perception, however ill conceived, may innocently get rooted as the hard truth, and takes up a dominant position rock-hard in their belief system. The bereaved will then defend it wholesomely as the only truth for they and the whole world to accept. The weight of sadness paralyses the ability to be logical. On one hand, they wish to be left alone doing nothing at all to contain the sadness. On other hand, they want to be seen able to deal with the funeral and move on in life. On one hand, they want to cry alone over their own sorrow and on the other hand, they assume that they are expected to please the visitors, often agreeing with advices, suggestions and demands from other people, which they may regret later on. Delayed regrets can raise delayed questions about their integrity, for they have gone against their own wishes and probably the wishes of the deceased, which cannot be undone. It will generate guilt and inadequacy, turning a harmless grief into a harmful one.

When questions are asked, answers have to be provided. Loaded with deep sorrow, paralysed by that hurt, bombarded with too many questions, which demand instant answers, the grief stricken person is dropped into an impassable state. To add fuel to the fire, many questions are unanswerable requiring medical knowledge or Godly powers. The bereaved need to stand still in order to get all the answers to all the questions before moving on in life. The living life cannot stand still; it is like a constantly moving escalator. They cannot halt at the time of the death taking time to find all the answers. In reality they have to move on in life. Therefore anyone trapped in that situation will be pressurised by himself or herself to make up some answers to solve that problem quick and easy. The greatest danger of the quickly and easily fix is that the bereaved would do it in secret. The *answers* produced in that kind of context, whether the answers are correct or not, will automatically progress through a cascade of inevitable evolution into the "*whole truth*" and nothing but the *unshakable truth as perceived by the bereaved* as illustrated by the following case.

A lady patient who was treated for long standing harmful grief generated by her "storming out" of her mothers house after a heated quarrel in relation to the lady's choice of partner. On arrival at her destination, she was informed that her mother had died of a heart attack. She immediately returned to the death scene. She hugged the body of her mother with unstoppable tears. She could not let the body be removed by the funeral directors, causing many hours of delay for the funeral. The question that she asked in *her own mind* on her way to the death scene was "Did my quarrel and storming out cause my mother's death?" In *her own mind* she made the answer, "Yes, I caused her death." She never told her *"truth"* for thirty years and she suffered harmful grief, in the form of feeling unworthy, making sacrifices, and lacking in energy and ambitions. During the therapy, it was revealed that her mother had suffered from serious vascular disease, which could have caused her heart attack anytime without the need for any kind prompting. Even though she had prior knowledge of her mother's pre-existing condition the strength of her sadness effectively ignored the facts and she held on to her *"truth"* for thirty years and that was until she received the treatment from KKA.

First the *answers* will take the status of the ultimate truth, and then they become embedded in their belief as the righteous one. Therefore the *answers* will be believed as the *"ultimate facts"*. The second step will be the *ultimate facts* passing a judgment with a verdict of *"someone is guilty of something"*. Inevitably the verdict of *"guilty"* will then get attached to the *"ultimate facts"*. Because the bundle of the *guilty verdict* and the *ultimate facts*, which are almost always based on assumptions. It is important to take account that those assumptions are evolved within the boundaries of the secret thoughts solely connected with the death of a loved one. The assumptions metamorphosed to *ultimate facts* are reinforced as the bereaved holds another belief that they are the only persons responsible to uphold love, justice and respect to the deceased. Inevitably but spontaneously, strong feeling of anger and hate come to occupy their mind. It soon becomes the most dominant and provoking thoughts during the entire waking time, literarily taking over their life. It is all because love and justice amalgamated with the sadness of the *"never to return departure"* of their loved one. According to the law of God and all humans from time immemorial all guilty persons need to embrace some degree of punishment and there shall not be any exemptions.

Automatically as the third step in the evolution of harmful grief, it receives the stamp of punishment. There it will stay as the unquestionable and absolute truth or the right thing to do for the rest of their life.

If the guilty party is the bereaved themselves, they have to install the punishment by themselves. Because the whole package of the *questions* and their answers followed by the *ultimate facts* and the *judgement of guilt* based on the *ultimate facts* are solely and squarely built upon the foundation of extreme love and the proportionate loyalty towards the deceased. The self-punishment has to be on a scale of absolute fairness to the maximum imaginable level of that love and loyalty. There are no units of measurement in this situation, everything is manufactured by pure assumptions by the bereaved, what kind of punishment is fair and how much of it is the maximum.

Completely unaware of the above process as described, the bereaved falls into the trap of filling with self-sacrifice and emotional sufferings as pennants in everyday of their life. Paradoxically, they carry on suffering and wondering what is happening to them, which everyone, including them, fails to fathom the reasons for their suffering. Especially, as time passes on they believe grief cannot be the cause for their troubles, because by that time they are expected to be doing and feeling all right according to the traditional beliefs. The *harmful grief* is born and it can happen straight after the death or may appear any time after in their life.

On the other hand if the guilty party happens to be another person, the bereaved will raise untold anger and hatred towards those persons. The anger and hatred evoked associated with grief may have valid reasons or it can be based on ill-conceived information influenced by personal and social/tribal beliefs. As mentioned above, the same dynamics of love and fairness towards the dead have to be upheld. The dead cannot be brought back to deal with the questions and therefore the anger and hatred cannot have an end. The bereaved will see any attempt by anyone else to reinterpret, as perceived by them as the reality, *the ultimate facts plus the judgement of guilt* as incorrect or unwarranted as an attack on their integrity, love and respect towards the deceased. The bereaved will vehemently resist any such attempt even from the professionals. Any appeal to reopen the debate will evoke fresh pain to the bereaved and the process will be perceived as most arduous. Therefore as far as the bereaved is concerned it is best left alone in status quo. Continuous harbouring of the never-ending hatred and anger will drain mental energy and upset the metabolic and immune system of the bereaved. They will start suffering from both perceptional/behavioural malfunctions and physical illnesses. The outcome would be that the bereaved has to suffer from the *harmful grief* in whatever form it may manifest on top of the loss of the loved one, who might have been the king pin balancing the happiness or contentment in their life so far.

Cultural, social and religious dogmas and family values influence the nature of some of the questions, but never is the compelling force. The immense sorrow from the loss of the loved one always remains as the centrepiece of how the questions are fashioned. The only way any human being can respond to the simultaneous onslaught of sadness and the questions raised following the death is often by the sufferer innocently forced to manufacture some answers. *The phenomena described above, in the opinion of KKA, forms the dynamics of harmful grief. Therefore harmful grief is nothing to do with anything else other than to do with unanswered or wrongly assumed answers to the many spontaneous but inevitable questions which are raised at the time of death of a person.*

Sadness or sorrow from a loss, namely grief, becomes harmful because the chain reactions of questions-answers-judgments-verdicts of guilty generate negative emotions demanding punishments. In fact, the bereaved faithfully believe it is the righteous thing to do. Holding on to the negative feelings towards oneself or towards others, is equally self-damaging, by the simple fact, that harbouring and processing such emotions takes a heavy drain on their energy. They assume it is a cross to bear to their grave and nothing can be done in tandem with the loss, which is irreversible. To make matters worse, they might even believe that forgiving or forgetting the wrongs is disrespectful and insulting to the love, which they hold towards the deceased. The last thing the bereaved will ever suspect that their grief could be the prime cause for their somatic illness, which seemingly fails to respond to all the conventional treatments. It is also common when one illness is treated a new problem will take the place of the previous illness, frustrating the patient and the medical team alike. There is no escape or choice in such predicaments, but to suffer. The hurting process is different from the feeling of sadness or sorrow. It progresses into physical malfunctions and/or emotional turmoil, which can masquerade as any known illness and that, is what harmful grief can do to anyone.

The seeds of harmful grief may be sown immediately after the death. This is a major difference from all previous stipulations how grief establishes. In some people those seeds are nipped before it takes root to grow, directing the grieving process into a harmless one. There is no general pattern for the time it may take to neutralise those seeds or to stop the grief from changing into a harmful one. On the other hand, the seeds may germinate within seconds or at least within hours after death, taking root and growing to cause hurt and injury as previously described resulting in harmful grief. On the other hand, it may take an unpredictable number of days to have the conversion into harmful grief depending upon how soon the bereaved had time or strength to complete the questions and the answers.

The process of turning grief into a harmful grief is potentially dangerous, as it is most likely to culminate in punishment of some kind such as breaking up relationship, inciting vengeful activities towards the hated person or persons. This hatred can even extend to terrorism, war and global destruction. The history is full of such events and will continue to happen. KKA sincerely hopes that this book may avert some of them, if only one.

Single session treatment of grief using Question & Answer model for a complete resolution.

Important house rules-
A grieving person is carrying a huge burden of sorrow and what they expect from the professionals or anyone else who would set upon helping them is simply help, help and help, from the word go. Questions like "what can I do for you?" or "how can I be a help?" will put the responsibility of identifying the problem and choosing the kind of help required back on to the patient. It can be very irritating to them because they cannot identify the problem or the need. Constructing a rapport from the very first moment of contact is highly essential for any kind of fruitful outcome of the treatment.

The bereaved carries a lot of hurt. They are expecting help from the word go. They cannot and will not take any comments, especially patronising, which would infer criticism or judgments on their already well rooted *answers and verdicts* as described above. At the beginning, the therapist has to accept in its totality whatever views the patient brings with them. Patients neither will be able to accept nor it will make any change in their beliefs with statements such as 'that is not true', 'that is silly', 'that is not how it works', 'that person is not wrong', 'he/she was right, you know', 'it is time you started thinking otherwise', 'you will forget in time', 'think only the good things', 'stop thinking things like that', 'time will cure all that', 'you will get over it'. The worst thing is telling them what they have to do, like 'that is what the dead person would want you to do'. The therapist has to work outside those commonly spoken clichés. Any corrections should wait until beliefs and opinions are changed in their on mind, after listening to the therapist's explanations and philosophies. The entire discussion must remain ***totally neutral and non-judgemental.***

The spoken words and especially the body language need to be carefully chosen, as more than the therapist observing the patient, the patient will be picking up every little expression the therapist will make. Smiling in the wrong context may offend the patient, even when the therapist knows some of their statements are outrageously unrelated or wrong. One way the therapists can express total neutrality is by openly telling the patient, that they are not there to take sides or pass judgement on anything. The patient will be reassured that the therapist will give only factual explanations related to what has happened. The therapist has to spell out that their vast experience and training to explain how the professionals and the system work. The explanations that they would give are not meant to justify or condemn the actions of any party, including the bereaved and the deceased. The therapist can make provisions to alter the affects using imagery and metaphor to help to discharge the anger or the guilt. Therefore every comment has to be framed as explanations, and not to be seen as judgment and verdicts. Through such explanations, as described at length later, the patient can be directed or guided to relinquish his or her anger or guilt, without the need to ridicule, punish or put anyone down.

Many bereaved would say that they suffer from a feeling of emptiness. One patient said 'It is as if a forest fire burnt everything; nothing is visible or tangible; there are just heaps of the same coloured (monochromatic) ash wherever I look'. One could use the same metaphor in therapy. While talking to a person in grief for the first time, the therapist can often build quick rapport if they can suggest an identical feeling that they might be suffering from, such as 'You *may (not 'will' or 'are')* be feeling empty, like one bereaved had expressed to me her inside feeling is like a forest after a fire'. Mentioning identical feelings is not the same as sharing. It is important not to express in any form that the therapist is able, or wanting, to share their grief, simply because grief by its very nature is absolutely unique and private. For example statements such as "I know how you feel", "I share your hurt/sadness" will damage rapport. KKA believes that almost all the bereaved would believe that nobody could ever understand how he or she is feeling and certainly does not want to share his or her very personal grief.

Though their feelings are uniquely theirs and can never be experienced by anyone else, however, what KKA would say to them would be something like this: "I need some way of understanding how you feel. Even though I can never really understand exactly how you feel, however from my vast experience of listening and helping many people with grief I will be able to interpret your feelings. Therefor everything that you will tell me can help me to help you". Very often they will feel free to outpour the unvented negative thoughts originated by the loss. Up until then they might have been hoarding those thoughts and had not told anyone.

First step in the treatment – *identifying the needy patient and giving appointment*

One single session can transform the life of a person who has been living with harmful grief, irrespective of how long and how bad they were suffering. Any suspicion of grief, which might be influencing the presenting illness, KKA will express openly to the patients, about the possibility of grief contributing in the dynamics of their illness. When the patients talk about the loss of someone, their body language is observed for hurt and sadness, or even weeping overtly. The issue is confirmed by directly asking "do you feel upset, angry or sad while you are talking about that person, right now?" If the answer is yes, KKA carries on with the treatment package then and there or gives an appointment within a week, because the emotion has been stirred up and turned 'hot', and it requires urgent intervention. They will be explained that the therapy will need only one session lasting one to one and half hour, and it will help them very much. There is no need to explain any further, because the very explanation constitutes most of the treatment itself. KKA also tells them that only good things will happen when the therapy session ends. He also reassures them that he will be guiding them all the away through the entire session, giving full support and strength for them to go through it.

The second step – *choosing which grief to start with*

The patient will be invited to talk freely about the deceased, and the details of the circumstances when they died. If there is more than one death compounding the presenting grief, after taking details of all the deaths, finally by mutual agreement choose one death, which the patient thinks the most active. Generally they go for the loss of the person, who was the dearest. KKA likes to confirm it directly with the patient by asking which one is (not *was*) most hurtful? The patient will then be assured that it is important to deal with the most grieving one first, at same time reassuring that all the other deaths will be dealt with later.

The third step – *introduction of metaphors to the patients*

a) *The boat metaphor for life*
KKA introduces this metaphor by telling the bereaved that, "I would like to tell you a metaphor for you to consider. It is a philosophical attempt to understand the beginning and the end of our life. It has enabled many people to re-position their views on matters of life and death. Through that modelled vision of life, they were helped enormously to come in terms with their loss of a loved one". KKA pauses a little and carries on as if the listener is just as keen to hear it, just as much as KKA is to tell them.

The same metaphor has helped many people, who have been faced with terminal illness. From the first moment anybody is informed that their illness is incurable, it tips them into severely disabling anxiety making their life and the life of their contacts very unpleasant and dark. The boat metaphor helps not only to remove the preoccupation of death in the terminally ill as well as in their contacts, but also turn them around to look forward to spending their life more productively and contentedly.

"Imagine, we are put in a boat at the precise moment when our life begins. What I mean when we start our life in our mother's womb and not the time when we are born. During the time of ten months in our mother's womb, we make all the preparation, in other words growing and developing, which is necessary to enable us to come out and sail in the wide world, in other words, to live in the outside world. Imagine, the world is a large ocean. Just imagine, that we are already put in a boat while we are growing inside our mother's womb and we are acquiring everything, which is needed to launch and sail in that wide ocean. One day we decide to come out of our mother's womb. With the help of our mother we make our way out. That means we are born into the wide world and straight away we start sailing our boat all by ourselves.

All the people on the earth are sailing forward in a straight line and level with each other across that ocean. The newly born joins a new line level with all the others and carries on sailing side by side of the parents and siblings. Life cannot stop or stand still. Whether we are sleeping or rushing about, all of us would be travelling at the same speed and covers the same distance. We all have the same 24 hours in a day. No one can have one second more or one second less, and so also none of us can go any faster or slower than the others. In the usual sailing, you start from one port and sail in any direction you like and take the boat back to same port or any other port. However in this metaphor as it reflects your life, you start in your mother's womb, and you can only sail in one direction and that is straight forward all the time and nonstop until you reach your final port, when you have to say goodbye to everybody and leave the world. Most importantly, the truth remains that from the time we start our life inside our mothers womb, everyone sails his or her own boat by himself or herself. Nobody else can be in that boat nor sail anyone else's boat. Only you can take it to your final port. There is a specially designated port for you and me like everyone else. When you reach your port you have to stop. In other words, you have ended the journey of your life. Everybody has to do it and there is no exception.

When we all sail our own boats we do that at the same precise speed as all the rest, so that the tips of all the boats are levelled in a line drawn across the wide ocean. It so happens, at least to start with, you like most of us, will be sailing having your mum and dad sailing on either side close to your boat. Other people may be sailing far away form you. During your journey, some of them might move away from you and some one else will take the empty space. Perhaps the people who had moved away might come back to sail close to you again. Some of co-sailors will reach their designated port and they will say goodbye to us. Some one else move into their slot or it may remain empty. If we catch a lot of fish on our journey, we can share it with others. While we are sailing side-by-side we can express our love to one another, on other hand we might shout at each other in anger. Still no one can sail your boat and at the same time you cannot sail other's boats under any circumstance.

When we reach the designated port we have to stop sailing. Whether we like it or not we have to leave our boat. We have to say goodbye to others, who will continue to sail until they find their designated ports. Nobody can know where their specific port is, until the last second of their journey. One thing is sure that you cannot miss it, it will be very clear to you when you are there. Not only that you will know it is your port, but also your boat will stop. Nothing you could do apart from to say goodbye to the rest of the people and leave the boat. When you reach the port you have to stop the journey. Another truth is that, even if the boat is in good shape, in other words you are in good health, and only positive things has happened in your life, when you reach your port, you have to stop the journey, say goodbye and leave the boat. On other hand, even the entire boat is broken up and only one plank left, struggle you must, however hard it might be, somehow even by wading with one arm, you have to take your boat to your specially designated port. No way can you abandon the boat, before you reach the port, nor can you move one dot of a distance beyond?"

It is not uncommon that the bereaved believes that the deceased person used to take care of them, implying the dead person was sailing their boat. Since the departure of the loved one there is no one to sail their boat, forcing them to feel that they have become helpless and incapable to go on. They loose confidence to progress with life. This metaphor makes them to realise that, in reality, they were sailing their boat (life) all the time, which gives their confidence and independence back.

b) *The book in heaven metaphor for the 'why' and the 'right time' to die?*
KKA has had hardly any bereaved, who did not ask 'why him or why her', 'why it didn't happen to me, instead of him or her and 'why now'?

As soon as the boat metaphor is finished KKA will launch straight into "the book in heaven metaphor".

"My grandmother used to tell me a story. It is incredibly close to the reality of life and death. Once upon a time, in a little village one man called 'Agadhan' had a special pass to go to heaven and hell whenever he pleased. On regular trips he used to convey messages between the people in the village and their deceased friends and relatives, who have gone to live in heaven or hell, like the grandfather who died at the age of eighty-five with flu, the five year-old son who died with meningitis, the aunty who died in an accident etc. He was free to roam anywhere in the hell and heaven as he chose. After one of his regular trips as usual, the villagers gathered around him asking questions about their relatives and friends. In the middle of his download he told them how he came across a very large book in one of the largest rooms in heaven. All our names are entered in that book. Against each name there are only just two entries. The first entry is the precise second when our lives begin, and the other is the exact second when we die."

The chief of the village, who was listening very carefully, wanted to know "how do we know it is time to die?"

Agadhan answered, "Well, two messengers from God will come, and tell you that it is time for you go with them. The reason for two of them coming is to double check the exact time, as they have no authority to take you away one second earlier or one second later; and there never had been any mistake. I have never seen any mistake or alteration in the entries in the book, and there is no provision to do so if some mishap happens, meaning there is no room for errors."

The chief wanted to know, "What would happen if they miss the time of appointment."

Agadhan answered, "Then you will become immortal. There is no provision for rewriting the time of death."

The chief asked Agadhan, "When you go next time, please look up 'the times' against my name".

Agadhan took a special trip next day solely to look up the time for chief to die. Returning from his visit, as usual the villagers gathered around Agadhan. He told the chief in front of everybody "You are not going to believe this. I couldn't believe it either. So I doubled and triple checked and it is absolutely correct. It is only one month left before you will be called. In fact, it is precisely 2pm on Wednesday in four weeks time".

In utter disbelief and shock the chief wailed, "I am only forty-five years of age, never had an illness; I have been good to all; have not done any sin, and *why* God is doing this to me?"
Agadhan answered, "I am afraid, the time you started your life and the time you will die are entered. Once the entry has made, even God cannot change it. It is nothing to do with what you have done in you life".

The chief began to think seriously, and asked, "Can they (the messengers from God) pass thorough thick wall?"

"No, but they can come through if air or light can get through, even if it is only a crack, or a keyhole." Agadhan clarified.

The chief immediately ordered to build a room of twenty feet long, 10 feet wide and ten feet high in size, with two inches thick steel walls and with only a small door for entry. Once the door was locked from inside, no one would be able to open from outside, and it would become air and light tight. He decided to go inside the room on Monday, two days in advance and to stay till Friday that is two days after the time of death has passed. He put a mattress in the middle to sleep and arranged the food for four days in the order of breakfast, lunch and dinner around the mattress. He set a large vessel in the right hand corner to use as a toilet. He had to do everything in pitch darkness. He went inside on Monday lunchtime and shut the door from inside and settled down for the four days' stay of his lifetime. He could not light candles, as it would use up all the oxygen. He settled down. He ate his dinner; went to bed and slept; got up and went to the toilet; had breakfast, lunch and dinner; went to bed and slept. On Wednesday afternoon he touched his body all over and shouted, "Yes I am alive. I have beaten God. I am immortal. I have done something nobody had ever done before."

He was not going to take any chances just in case there was some last minute change or a mistake on someone's part. So he stayed inside as previously planned for anther two days. He came out on Friday afternoon, triumphantly, shaking his fists high up in the air and grinning from ear to ear. As soon as he opened the door, there were two messengers from God standing right at door. They told him, "Sir, it is time for you to leave this world. We came to take you to heaven."

The chief protested strongly and pushed the messengers aside saying "You can't touch me. You are late by two days. So you better leave without me and don't bother to come back."

But the messengers insisted that that they were on the correct time and there was no mistake. The furious chief turned to Agadhan and accused him, "You made a mistake or did you deliberately told me the wrong time? You all are liars and cheaters".

Agadhan and the people gathered shook their head and said, "There is no mistake on our part. This is the right time as written in the book."

The confused, angry and sad chief muttered, "Is it not Friday afternoon?" In unison, they all shook their heads and said, "No, it is Wednesday 2.pm precisely on the sundial!" When the penny dropped the chief collapsed at the feet of the two messengers. He had lost count of the days because he was in total darkness. In those days the only way to tell the time was by means of a sundial. It so happened he opened the door and came out at the correct time that was written in the book.

We all have a set time when our life on this earth will come to an end and that time is the moment of our death or "time-to-die". Leading to the time of death, one of the many things might happen, like a serious illness or some one might do a lethal mistake, or a tree falls on our head, or a natural disaster might happen, etc., etc. We all would remark that those events caused the death or killed the person. The reason we all think like that is because death of any kind and at any time is not acceptable to us. We are looking for something or someone to blame for the death. Such rationalisation inherently makes 'death' avoidable and so *"not inevitable"* at least, at that precise time to the precise person from that precise cause. The inevitability of death must be for someone else, at some other time and due to some other cause; but it shouldn't be the time or cause for that person who just happened to die. The naked fact is that, every one of us has to die and so death is inevitable. People say that if those so-called events did not occur, the person would have been still alive. But nobody asks the question of "precisely how long they would have lived?" There are millions of anecdotes of how people survive against all the odds and they die of something trivial, or some people just keel over unexpectedly and die. So let us accept that it is the 'time-to-die', which determines when we would die and not because what has happened preceding the death. If it was not for that particular cause of events preceded that death, something else would happen, and that death would happen anyway. Think about the fate of the village chief in the above story. *We cannot escape from death nor change the time when it will happen. There are only two goal posts in anyone's life. They are the time we start our life and the other the time we will die. Those goal posts are pre designated, in philosophical terms, which is non-negotiable and non-alterable. Let us believe in such a philosophy, which is very evident in the real history of mankind. It will give us a lot of answers to the question of why him or her?*

On the other hand, if it is not the time-to-die, one will survive through all the odds, even from a bullet. Being a doctor and witnessing many deaths, in spite of all scientific training, KKA believes in the fate of everyone having a time-to-die and that goalpost can never be moved. In the same way the goalpost of the time we start our life cannot be shifted by us. We do not have any control or power to alter, nor to ask for the 'time-to-start' or the 'time-to-die' in our life. Philosophically speaking there is no ultimate answer apart from the book in heaven model to the question of "what caused the death?" and "why at that particular time?" Even in homicide or suicide, it can be questioned. What caused the "cause?" Or what created the "cause"? What determined the "precise time"? The questioning can go on and on until we will end up in an answer, "if we were not born we could not die". So let us not talk about the cause of death, or the time when it occurs. Both have to happen without being neither asked for nor determinable by us.

The boat metaphor and the book in heaven metaphor have been found very beneficial and comforting when death is imminent in serious illnesses like cancers and other terminal diseases. Also the relatives may be introduced to the model of how grief can turn into causing harm and encourage them to ask question during terminal illness processes. KKA has had used these ideas in all these cases with huge benefit in the prevention of harmful grief.

Everybody treated for grief by KKA had no difficulty in accepting his philosophy. Moreover there is a high chance of some of the questions related to the cause of death, and certainly about the timing of death, which had been troubling their thoughts all along, to disappear instantly. Almost certainly the question "Why" would never need to be repeated. The patients would appear more relaxed after listening the above two metaphors.

c) The elastic band metaphor

Many patients have remarked about their everyday feelings following bereavement, that they have lost half of their self along with the loss of their loved one. Since the death of the loved one, they have been carrying a belief that they are incomplete or not full anymore; which automatically and involuntarily affects their ability to perform fully. KKA brings another metaphor to enlighten that problem. "The life has to move on like being on a non-stop conveyor belt, at the same time one cannot leave the death scene without solving all the unfinished issues. So, metaphorically, we solve the impossible by dividing ourselves into two halves. We then leave one half of our self at the scene of death, supposedly for that half to stay put until all the answers to all the questions are found, while the other half moving on with life. You may feel like that you are tied by an elastic band to the scene of death, looking back so often, to see what that half of you is doing. Nothing possibly could be done because it is frozen in time. You are stuck in that predicament as the life moves on while the elastic band is getting stretched, increasing the suffering." Usually the patients identify their predicament with the elastic band metaphor and it is worth telling them at this stage, so that when the treatment package is finished, they automatically will know that from that moment (the end of the session) they are free to move on in life feeling full, without being tied to the past.

e) *Fourth step – introducing the dynamic of harmful grief to the patients, that is the "Question and Answer Model©™", which may be a contributory factor to the cause of the illness, as well as to the resistance to treatments so far.*

The discussion with bereaved would start like this - "When some one very dear to you dies, it strikes deep into your heart. You are dazed, confused and feeling very sad. Your mind will be filled with a million questions about so many things from the past, the present and the future immediate and distant. It is basic human nature to ask a lot of questions at the time of any catastrophe or tragedy, which death is both. It is an essential part of the survival strategy, built into our DNA over the past millions of years of human existence. So every one, not just you will ask many questions."

KKA will then explain the intricate nature of how a harmful grief would take shape, as described below, in a language measured to suit individual patients, giving full opportunity for them to intervene and ask questions.

From now on KKA will use the name of the deceased instead of "loved one" during the interview. For the benefit of the book KKA will refer to deceased as "John".

"What I am going to talk about now is all about how you happened to suffer from grief because of all those questions, which had passed through your mind from the very moment of your realisation of your John's death. You have been asking those questions relentlessly even to this very moment, you and I are talking about it. It is important that you understand fully everything I will say. I will use simple terms of conversation and I hope that you will be able to follow my talk effortlessly. Please, there is no need for you to observe any formality, meaning please do interrupt, even in the middle of a sentence, stop me and ask me to explain again and again until you understand everything. I will explain using metaphors and other means. There are many ways of explaining the same thing and I am very experienced in doing that. The reason for this promise is that the successful outcome of our work and the ultimate help, which I assure you that you will get, wholly depends upon your grasp of what I am going to say."

"The questions, which most of the bereaved usually ask, are normally in the form of inquisitions for anything which could have been done by various people including yourself, or anything which happened differently, would have prevented the death itself or at least postponed the time of the death. More importantly, it could be about something, that was done or said by anyone causing great upset or un-necessary suffering to the deceased, during the period of illness leading to the death and around the funeral. Even in the cases of deaths, which were long expected and assumed to be acceptable, most often the same questions with the same gravity may be asked. It might not necessarily be a serious or grave issue. Instead it could be quite a trivial misbehaviour or attitude by others or by you, which happened to fall short of absolute politeness or decency or even just how it might have been perceived as disrespectful towards John. Such perception will only take possession of your thoughts, only when the questions being asked inside your mind just after the death had occurred or straight after the funeral. It will be highly charged with negative emotions. The severity of the offending deed or remark is usually disproportionate, distorted or even assumed compared to the reality, because of the intense sadness over the death rules all your feelings and judgement."

"The other kind of questions you might have asked would be thoughts about something wrong you or someone else had committed towards the dead person sometimes in the past, but did not do anything about it because you did not consider it as serious enough to act upon at the time when it was done. However, when extreme sadness strikes as you lost John, it is inevitable that you, for that matter anybody, would look back through memory for matters of that nature. Many things would have fled through your memory, in fact everything in you knowledge, which had happened related to John. Such recall of the 'not so important matters' in the past will transform them into 'matters of unforgivable guilt, anger, hate and resentment', again distorted by your grief."

"The problem with that kind guilt and many of the other previously described negative emotions, such as anger, hate and resentment, will be transformed or perceived by you as extremely serious. Though the original incident might have been trivial in reality or they might have been justifiably true in their validity such interpretations would be experienced in the your thoughts as solid reality, meaning nothing should or could change such interpretations. Instead they would become rock hard beliefs. Automatically, in other words you would not had any control or even understanding of what was happening, those beliefs almost instantly get stamped with a 'guilty verdict'. The process of 'guilty verdict' had to be concluded straightaway so that you would be freed from sorting out the most upsetting issues, so that you would have more time and energy to deal with many other immediate things such as organising the funeral and so on. One of most serious aspects of those 'guilty verdicts' is that they will become the final verdicts, partly because it is not possible to explain or apologise to your departed as he/she is dead and so he/she cannot give any form of reply either. The other reason for putting the seal of 'guilty verdict' as final, almost like writing in stone, is the grieving person, that is you, had to sort out a hundred and one things immediately following the death. Within the same slot of time you had to hold extreme and unprecedented sadness in your heart, and naturally you could not find time for a detailed re-thinking or critical analysis of the 'guilty verdict'. Any guilty verdict therefore will automatically demand reproach or punishment such as to create anger, hate or resentment towards the person who is guilty, often directed to oneself. It is easy to take the blame unquestioned on oneself. I call those issues as 'unfinished, or unanswered questions' meaning not properly and thoroughly dealt with. Commonly the 'guilty verdict' falls on someone who is perceived as not showing enough love towards John."

"I want you to take plenty of time and please have another look at what kind of questions passing through or even filling your thoughts immediately after the death of your loved one. On top of all those questions showering your thoughts, you were also required to deal with the funeral. At the same time you had to talk to so many people who would be coming to pay respect to the deceased. Naturally you wanted to be very polite and fair to everyone and making sure nobody was left out from your attention. While all those very busy activities had to be taken care off, you were also trying to answer all those questions, which had been continuously popping into your mind. Within that kind of context, people have only two options to respond to those questions, either by giving the seemingly right answers or by shelving it for the time being to deal with some other time. During the early stages of grief no one is capable of thinking logically, practically or reasonably; paradoxically one believes that he or she is doing so. The tragedy of that is the answers produced become written in stone, permanently, with a verdict of guilt on someone's part. As it is easy to blame oneself, because nobody else can question it or disapprove it, and the whole process of questioning and answering has got to be done very quickly, because of innumerable other duties to be carried out, the entire process is conducted secretly in the minds of the person who is grieving. Rightly or wrongly he or she becomes loaded with guilt. The 'self-locking' process then takes on. The bereaved becomes so ashamed or wanting to be punished for their perceived 'crime' towards the dead. The guilt, thus created will be locked away secretly, unabated in their every day thoughts and will be reminded and reflected in their minute-by-minute life. Creation of such negative feelings either towards themselves or to other persons and the continued harbouring those feelings will convert grief into 'harmful grief'."

On the other hand, if the answers manufactured entirely in the thoughts of the bereaved failed to develop any negative emotion, the grief will remain simply as a 'harmless one'. It is not uncommon that harmful answers may be converted to harmless one at a later date due to the secondary self-analysis, or receiving further understanding from sources not available earlier. **It is most significant that an established harmless grief will never turn into a harmful grief.**

KKA believes that, the initiation of the process of determining, which grief would turn into a harmless grief or a harmful grief takes place at the very beginning of the bereavement. However, when dealing with harmful grief, irrespective of whether their initial interpretations had been changed or not, it is most important to bring them all up, one by one and neutralise them if necessary.

KKA repeats the assurance of expert guidance and absolute support to the patients by informing them that, "discussing the already explained issues between us, utilising my experience and expertise, and what I have learned from treating grief in many people; together we will be able to convert all the harmful answers into completely harmless."

"You might have left some of the questions unattended or unanswered, because only the dead person could have answered them. Some of the questions unanswered might be because they involve medical or other technical matters, which you did not have the training to understand. Or it might be because it was not possible at that time to receive a trustworthy and full explanation due to the unavailability of an expert or a professional source. Also it might be simply because you were so much involved in carrying out many other jobs, which naturally should take priority, you did not have time to give a satisfactory answer and as you had moved on with your life those questions were put in a drawer and even forgotten. All the questions, even if they may appear to you as trivial or unconnected to grief, need addressing. You and me working together, using my training in medicine and expertise in human behaviour, we need to and we will provide every one of those questions with answers, which will neutralise all the existing negative emotions. We can sort all of them right now. There is no need to leave anything at all behind. Especially any question, which were connected or concerned with the dead person (using the real name of the dead person), with wrongful answers or unanswered and they could only be settled with your departed, but you did not have the opportunity to do so, all of those issues had to be mentioned and dealt with right now. I will help you all the way. It is my expertise to find the real and proportionate answers, which you will be surprised to find wholly acceptable, meaning you would no longer feel any guilt or anger over those issues. Some of the issues justifiably would have left great anger or guilt in you. Even those solid issues need to be neutralised, meaning I have many different ways to help you to get rid of the associated anger or the guilt completely. If you continue to hold on to any of the negative emotions inside you, however small, will damage your wellbeing beyond any doubt. It is not fair on the top of the sadness that you are already enduring from the loss of your loved one, that you are further harmed by the negative feelings, such as anger, hatred, guilt and shame. What is important at this moment is to obtain full neutralisation of all harmful issues so that when we finish this session, you would be totally free from the harm that generated as part of your grief."

At the end of the above spiel, KKA invites the grieving person to open up with anything and everything, most certainly the unanswered and the unfinished issues. Taking issue by issue, including issues, which might clearly show wrongdoings by someone, he turns every single issue into harmless products. He extensively uses metaphors and imagery in explaining each event to give them a plausible alternative understanding or reasoning and effectively guiding the bereaved to create and freely accept a totally different verdict about what had happened. Naturally, the newly created meaning and verdict would be neutral, in other words, without generating any negative emotions at all. Having the benefit of the time passed by after the demise of the loved one, during which many things might have happened and simply enlightening or reframing such events can throw new knowledge and so new understanding. Some of the issues could be easily neutralised of their harmful effect in that manner. All it would need is to draw their attention to it and that would remove

the associated negative emotions. In issues of real wrongdoing by someone who would have justifiably created negative emotions such as anger
and hatred, KKA has specially designed methods to neutralise the anger
and hate permanently. Some of the techniques are described below.

Most of the anger and hatred generating incidents are something,
which happened during the last illness leading to the death or at the time
of the funeral. However it is not unusual when tragedy occurs, people
make journeys into the past forgotten events and reinstate them as fresh
issues with more vigorous scrutiny. It is immaterial when it had happened, but it is important to address every issue in details and neutralise
the negative affect. The same techniques would apply to all.

After listening to the full contents, the first thing to do is to make corrections in the understanding of the details, especially misquotes or mis-
information about medical or technical issues. For example, one grieving
mother was asking the question in the case of a suicide committed by
her young son, who was in the army. He killed himself by firing his rifle
through his mouth. She was told that he was alive when they found him
and took him to the nearest casualty, where attempts were made to save
his life, but he died. The mother carried in her thoughts a doubt whether
there was something else, which the army wanted to hide from her. She
was under the firm belief that the death should have happened instantly
if someone had shot through his or her mouth. She also wanted to know
whether her son was conscious and suffered a great deal of pain. KKA
had personal experience of almost a similar case of a police person who
did exactly the same and was brought alive to the casualty while KKA was
on duty. The person was deeply unconscious even though he lived for a
while in the casualty receiving resuscitative procedures before he died.
Sharing such personal experience and telling her that her son would be
deeply unconscious from the start and so that he could not have felt any
pain before his death. More importantly for her to know that it was possible a person could be alive for a while after a lethal shot and the death

was inevitable. The mother was very relieved and all her negative emotions were neutralised.

Very often the anger or hatred is created by an action, which the bereaved believes in their opinion had caused undue suffering to their loved-one during the the last illness, either emotionally or physically often by the lack of adequate pain control. It might be an act of neglect, as perceived by them and not uncommonly derived from either false statement, lack of empathy and standard of care or inadequate and construed knowledge about some facts. The bereaved believes that such neglect either have caused a lot of pain or insulted the basic human dignity of a dying person. The majority of those beliefs are based on assumptions and once formed they become strong and unwavering beliefs. KKA has been told many times by the bereaved that "how could they do such a thing", "no way, under any circumstance, I cannot forgive them for that", "it is very cruel and wicked and inhumane to treat my loved one like they did", "they would not have done such a thing to an animal", and so on. All that would be needed to neutralise the negative emotions is to give simple, truthful and unbiased explanations to highlight the factual reality.

One of the common causes of self-guilt or anger creation is someone taking decisions against the wishes of the deceased at a time very close to their death. For example, the seriously ill mother wished or even insisted to die in her own bed at her own home. However the son could not bear to see his mother suffering and wanted to do the best for her, probably even to save her from dying. He decided she should be taken to hospital even against the wish of the daughter, who had argued that they should let the mother die at home. The son was convinced something positive could be done in hospital. The mother was admitted and died that night with no one there to hold her hand. The mother, in theory underwent all that trouble being transported and to be bedded in a strange place, the hospital and died "alone". The daughter was very angry towards the son and the son was very guilty, neither of them felt that there could be a reprieve to their feelings. On the other hand, the scenario could be the opposite. The deceased wanted to stay at home and refused to be sent to the hospital. The son agreed to the mother's wish against the wishes of some others. During the last few minutes or hours prior to the death, it was awful as their loved-one struggled to breath, choking and obviously very distressed. The guilt or anger develops based on an after thought or assumption that they should have ignored the wish of the mother and made her go to the hospital. She could have died peacefully. When grief strikes with extreme sadness, there is no right judgement, as everything could be argued either way and there could be always a different way to the one had been carried out.

Metaphor of God: - KKA uses the "metaphor of God" to neutralise guilt or anger formed in that way. Another scenario, which may create similar kind of guilt and anger, can happen when the bereaved happens to be attending the deceased very diligently most of the time. The death happens when the bereaved has just left the bedside to do something very essential or personal, or because they are told that the dying person is in a stable state. Sometime they are persuaded to go home for a short rest, which they really needed. In some cases the dying person them-selves persuade them to take a rest. The death happens just after they had left the bedside. The guilt and sadness in such cases are immense, which they would rate as unforgivable guilt for leaving the bedside and missing the goodbye.

KKA would start the metaphor. "Let us, for the time being believe the Biblical version of the creation of the world. God created the earth and all the creatures and vegetation, etc. etc. He created Adam, the human. He absolutely believed that he had created everything, which is required for the perfect world as far he is concerned. He did all that in six days and six nights because he was the almighty and knew everything and could do anything. He went to bed feeling very satisfied having done all the right things and feeling very proud of his creation. After a well deserved good night's sleep he woke up next morning and went round his 'perfect creation' for a second look. Then he saw Adam sitting on a rock looking all miserable and sad. When God asked the reason for his sadness and sulking look, Adam answered that he was feeling very lonely as he was the only human being on this wonderful world, even though he was told that he was created in the image God himself. What more could he expect? Adam revealed the real reason by explaining that he had no companion to share his life with. God realised his grave omission. He had used up everything and there was no unused material left to create another person. Admitting his shortcoming and apologetically he had to borrow a rib from Adam to create Eve as the companion to Adam."

"Even God could make mistake or was it a "mistake", as we all say always when something was not right, proper or adequate. The truth of the matter or the solid fact is that no one including God can only do something or anything at any one time, what one believes to be the right, the proper and the adequate at that precise moment in time. It is impossible for anyone to do anything other than what he or she, even God believes that to be the right thing to do at the time when the act is carried out. Afterwards or looking back, it turns out to be understood as "wrong" or a "mistake" and so on. The deed might be obviously the wrong thing in the perception of the rest of the world such as murder or pure neglect. At the time of the deed was committed, unknowingly or knowingly, that it might be seen as the wrong doing or neglect by the rest of the world, but the person who is committing that deed has to believe and will believe that it was the right and the best thing to commit. He or she could not have behaved in any other way, even if it meant that he or she deliberately wanted to do the wrong thing, but at that precise moment they had to believe that it was the right thing to do as far as they are concerned. It is the human bind and one needs to understand and accept, like Adam accepted the oversight by God and willingly offered his rib. So there is no such thing as committing a mistake in the eye of the committer because at that time they believed they were doing the right thing. Therefore they were incapable of committing anything else except what they believed as the right thing to do and so it never was a mistake at the time of its commitment. We can only be wise in the future and possibly avoid the same act again."

"Therefore it is not fair nor right to feel guilty over something that wasn't the appropriate act as judged after it was committed. When nothing can be labelled as a deliberate mistake, there is no need or place for guilt. In the case of God's shortcoming, neither Adam nor God were angry or felt guilty. Certainly God never was guilty. He just dealt with the situation and made up with what he needed to do, in other words he just made the correction and that was the end of the matter. There was neither never-ending analysis nor any persistent reminder of guilt or anger. If God could make "mistakes", who are we to judge anybody's mistakes? Let us understand things in its true perspectives. We often fall foul into the trap of instant reaction. By reconsidering the facts there is no need to hold on to the anger or guilt any more and once and for all let us throw away all the guilt and anger."

Most of the bereaved would be able to relinquish their guilt following the above philosophical enlightenment. Just in case if they continued to hold on to part of their guilt, they would be able to completely neutralise the guilt or anger during the occasion of "bidding goodbye" in the final part of the treatment when they would have the opportunity to apologise to the deceased, just like God apologised to Adam and that would be enough to wipe the last thread of their guilt.

It is not unusual in the experience of KKA to have a few bereaved people who could not forgive or stop feeling the anger or the guilt. They might even admit that they were convinced that there was no need for them to have such feelings. On the other hand, they simply could not let the guilt feeling go, which was ruling their life for a long time. It might be because they were so used to carrying those feelings and it was not easy to shake it off or they might require further convincing that the person who had acted badly did not have any other option within their belief or skill training. It is very difficult to persuade the bereaved to simply wash away the anger and hatred towards a third party, who had committed a very black and white wrong doing, which the world would acknowledge as wrong or even cruel. Any amount of forgiveness assisted by faith or by advice from close family or friends or even by professional therapists, they just could not stop hating or harbouring the anger. It is important that one-way or another, they have to know from their heart that they no longer feel even a trace of anger or guilt. It is also important to do the convincing by bringing in more metaphors and explanations. It will not work by simply telling them to stop feeling guilty or angry because no good would ever come of it, or they are wrong to hold on to their feelings. To uphold the rapport, it is paramount that the therapist must not judge them as wrong to form the guilt or anger. In fact one should applaud what they had done under the circumstances of extreme sadness, and instant reactions are fully justified. It had saved them from freezing in time and helped them to move on in life even if it were in a harmful way. Applying the same reason as in the philosophical metaphor of God making mistake, they also could not have helped from creating such negative emotions. However the time has come to get rid of them because such negative feelings have no place in their future life. KKA uses the following methods to help in such cases.

"Please, let us continue with our discussion in order to remove your anger completely, as it is making your life and possibly the life of others close to you very miserable and suffering. It is not fair for you to suffer not only from the loss of your loved one, but also continued to be punished because of someone else's wrongdoing. I will help you to get out of that shackle and make yourself free. At present the anger that you are harbouring is perfectly justified when it started. At the same time one needs to ask whether it is necessary to carry on, especially when you know that you cannot undo, what had been done and for worse, you are not in a position to correct it?

Sometimes the guilty party is very powerful and you might be feeling help-less to do anything about them, at the same time the anger towards them is only getting stronger. The stronger the anger gets or the more hatred bubbles in your thoughts, every minute of your life, the more you become dysfunctional and disabled to enjoy the pleasures of love and life."

THE 3 OPTION STRATEGY **to remove or neutralise the negative emotion like guilt, hate, anger or resentment towards another person or persons, in connection with the death of the loved one.**

KKA would take the bereaved through *three options* for them to con-template in the order as given below, because if they managed to clear their negative emotions in the first stage, there would not be any purpose to take them through the rest of the options.

Option 1. "For the sake of thinking through a different angle about what had upset you, I would suggest that you have to reverse the roll in your imagination. In other words, put yourself in their position. I would recom-mend that, for a short while, you really have to live through every step of the events being those persons. Please take as long as you want to re-enact that roll. It is also important to take full consideration of the circumstances, the skills, the training, the availability of resources, and all other possible knowledge of those persons who had committed the wrongdoings." After a few seconds silence – "Now tell me as best as you can the uncensored thoughts which had passed through your mind." Whatever had mentioned would be discussed fully as follows - " let us talk about how and what had made them take those particular actions at that particular time, which had turned out to be wrong and which had caused a lot of hurt and anger since then. Most probably they had done to the best of their ability as they could not have done anything else at that time."

KKA will expose and elaborate their ignorance and incompetence, which became the foundation of how and what made that offending event take place. It might be simply the lack of time or resources or even how little the scientific world could offer to do anything else. Then he will put his proposal to the bereaved - "If you can accept this new knowledge and concept, please forgive them for their ignorance at the same time wish them to become better, so that they might not hurt anybody in future." Very often many bereaved would accept and would be able to relinquish their own guilt or the anger and hatred towards the third party. Not uncommonly the bereaved might be angry with the deceased, because something the deceased did regarding the last illness such as disclosures of the nature of illness or noncompliance of medical advice, etc. KKA had found that the above approach of exposing and explaining the ill understood gaps works well in the majority of the cases.

Option 2.
In some cases the above option fails to remove the guilt or hatred, probably because the bereaved strongly believes that the third party had no reason what so ever to do such a wrong thing. Moreover, they believed that the offenders were capable of doing the appropriate things, but deliberately ignored as if they could not care less. Sometimes the wrongdoing was wilfully carried out as in wanton killing or wilful neglect leading to the death. With that kind of understanding, the guilt or anger would be very aggressive and as a norm and would require some form of reprisals or punishment. It is much worse when they had already made every effort to take reprisals, but failed for various reasons, especially when the culprits were very powerful and wilfully distorting facts. The guilt is also much higher in cases of suicide because the bereaved, as the closest kin, assumes that they should have paying more attention to what was happening to their loved one and done something to prevent the suicide.

KKA would start with reminding the metaphor "The book in Heaven" to underpin the predetermined time to die. In the same breath he would agree with the bereaved that their anger was the normal and natural reaction any human would feel, as one might say, fully justified against such a deed. However, if it were his/her time to die as one would like to believe, nothing could or would alter the exact time of death. The only different thing could have happened would be some other events could have happened prior to the time of death. Even in the case of wanton killing or freak accidents and even suicide or utter negligence, if those events or circumstances, which seemingly precipitated the death were not to happen, something else had to happen up to that precise moment of death and then they would take blame to cause the death. The person had to die at that precise moment and until the death happens something had to happen. Because the bereaved would be suffering badly from the harming effect of grief, in practice in the context of this therapy, almost all people would accept that the death was inevitable at that particular time.

When the bereaved rejected option one and just could not let the anger or guilt go, KKA would then ask them –" Please close your eyes if you could, simply because closing the eyes will help you to focus more intensely and to follow effortlessly, what I am going to suggest to you, right now. Everything that I will be suggesting will help you a great deal to neutralise or remove the anger that you have been holding on to so long. You may even want to agree with me, that it is time to let all the negative emotions, *for example the anger and guilt* go for good, because you are ready to turn your life around, back to normality and reclaim your fundamental right to be loved by others, to love others freely, and to en-joy the pleasures of the free flowing love and the life itself. You may also be thinking that you have suffered enough from someone else's wrong doings and it is time for you to pick a normal life, which you rightfully deserve. In order to do that, you have to wipe off all your anger and guilt completely and that is exactly what I am going to help you to achieve."

"Right, that is good. You have closed your eyes. In a moment, I will be asking you to imagine certain things. I want you to pretend as good and real as you can, putting all your heart into your imagination. It is beneficial if you are able to add a little of your own creative components or dreams into those imaginations. So please strongly immerse yourself in your imagination that you are reliving events, here and now."

" I want you cast your thoughts to those occasions, which caused all that anger/guilt in you. Taking all the time you need, I want you relive those moments, if necessary, going over and over until you experience the hurt or anger. Holding on to the feeling, I want you to analyse the scenario hard and realistically but adequately measured, not one bit less nor one bit over. Again taking time, think of a judgement or decision on what kind of reprisal or punishment to be given to that person. Take your time and let me know when you have formulated the proportionate action." *KKA waits for the answer.*

"Good. Right now, in your imagination, putting all your heart into it, please carry out everything that you want to do to that person without mincing any word or action. As you are doing everything in your imagination, you can fulfil all you would want to do. You can say things loudly or act outwardly, but do it exactly to your decision and repeat everything as many times as you need. Stop it only when you are really happy with the outcome and that will be when you do not need to hold on to even a shred of anger. Even though you are doing all the reprisal in your imagination, the effect will be the same as if you were doing it in reality, because you are putting all your heart into your imagination to make it real. You need to understand that what had happened to you was like a ball of fire, which burnt you, sometime ago. It hurt you then, very badly and you reacted with anger when it happened. The fire was put out a long time ago or it was just a one-off flame and so the actual burning process had also stopped a long time ago as well. But the reason you continued to feel the anger is because, you had an illusion that fire had not stopped and continued to hurt you. In other words, it was kept alive only as an illusion in your imagination and so another imagination of reprisal being carried out works absolutely and realistically with real benefit."

Nine out of ten people would be happy and contented with the removal of all their anger, guilt or hatred with the second option. The remaining cases, because they were so upset, would continue to feel that some part of that anger could not be reconciled. The third option would work in all the cases, because of the following reasons. The human brain can generate and experience only one kind of emotion at any given time or moment. Almost all of us believe that different kinds of emotions can co-exist, which is true as we experience them, but it is an illusion. In reality, they are not running simultaneously in parallel lines. In other words, when each type of feelings, for example sadness, anger, feeling good and feeling friendly are presented to our awareness they are cut into small segments and then interposed like the links of a chain made out of different emotional segments. Our brain is so inherently canny to do it in such a way that it is like watching a movie. The actions in a movie are recorded on the film in segments. When it is run faster it gives the illusion of the movements as unbroken and we do not experience it as segments. In the similar manner, when the emotional segments are presented to our awareness we have an illusion of experiencing different kind of emotions at the same time.

Option 3.
In the third option the above phenomenon is used to neutralise any negative emotions and remove them permanently within a very short time. The idea is to link the negative emotion with a positive emotion, every time a negative emotion is presented, in a way the positive emotion is actively and deliberately slapped on to the negative emotion, like a hammer hitting to crush something which is long overdue to be rid of. Creation and continued existence of negative emotions is always an active process because the dynamics of it requires analysis, judgement and execution

of the verdict and punishment, at least in the imagination. Therefore processing and upholding negative emotion demands the usage of high volumes of mental and physical energy, as everyone experiences tiredness as part and parcel of having negative emotion. On the other hand positive emotion is passive, almost like 'a default emotion' and one does not need to work on it. It just will be there as long as there is no negative emotion to override it. One of the commonest failures in the treatment of negative emotion is that some of the therapies are aimed to build positive emotion independently on top of the existing negative emotion, without neutralising the negative emotion, prior to establishing the positive emotion. The bereaved, for that matter anyone, would never be happy to carry on having negative emotions, bubbling up spontaneously or by deliberation, because it is always hurtful and destructive to him or her. The healthy survival of everyone requires contentment and good feeling. The human brain is tuned to accept a positive emotion and install it in place of a negative emotion, if and when the two are presented in tandem, provided the negative emotion has been at least weakened using the above mentioned options one and two.

It is obviously evident that in human behaviour when a person thinks or talks about a happy or joyful moment or incident, it is impossible for that person to do it without a smile on his or her face. Similarly it is impossible to describe a hurtful or anger provoking incident with a smile. He or she has to have a facial expression reflecting that negative emotion. The key factor in this third option is to ask the bereaved in their imagination to make a seemingly ridiculous or laughable statement. Every time when the bereaved remembers the causative incident they would experience anger towards the person who had caused it. However much the bereaved wishes and tries to get rid of the anger and hatred by forgiving the people who had caused it, they would fail. Forgiving, in practice, is almost like telling oneself to forget the whole thing. Everyone knows it will not go away from their thoughts. Moreover, because they would be repeating the recollection and debates of the offending deeds and the associated persons, whenever they try to re-move the negative emotions, it is more likely that the negative emotions could get stronger rather than to fade away. The third option overrides all such issues.

KKA would start the **Third Option;** by making a statement to the be-reaved that "It is apparent that you continue to experience anger/hatred when we talk about what happened. What they did was very wrong, whichever way anyone could look at it. No one could justify what was done and there are no excuses for acting the way they did. You are right to feel angry/hatred and no one could argue with the way you are feel-ing. On the other hand, what happened was in the past and was a one-off incident. You and I know that it cannot and will not happen again to your loved one or to you. The fact remains that what happened at that time was undoubtedly wrong and it had caused great upset and hurt. Undoubtedly it is continuing to cause hurt inside you every time you think about it because it is generating the emotion of anger/hatred, which we call negative emotions. At every occasion a negative emotion is gener-ated in your brain, in other words whenever you feel the active presence of the negative emotion, while you are going about with the routine of the day, it could be assumed that many harmful chemicals may be released into the general circulation as a result of that experience. Whether you like it or not every time the negative emotion surfaces it can release harm-ful chemical, which may be the root cause of many illnesses. Moreover you would remain unhappy and you have to set aside a lot your time, energy and effort controlling those negative emotions, leaving you with much less time and energy for your normal work and activities resulting in you becoming much less efficient in your everyday functioning. Because you will be underperforming you may start disliking yourself for being un-able to fulfil the expectations from your family and people connected with you. The dislike may soon become hate, which will be joined with anger and guilt for you letting others down. Then it will become a vicious cycle compounding your illness both physically and mentally."

"I would say that suffering like that is very unfair, as you have already suffered pain and hurt when it happened and you are continuing to suffer from someone else's wrongdoing. I would say that it is a double unfairness. You or anyone for that matter cannot undo what has happened already. But the carrying on with this on-going damage to you, affects not only your health and life, but also the health and the emotional wellbeing of the people attached to you. It is entirely caused through the continued generation of anger/hatred, which in all truth is created by you, in your thoughts. I am sure you will agree with me that it is time to put a stop to the creation of negative emotions."

"I know a way to achieve it and it had been very successful in many cases whom I have helped in the past. In fact this method, which I am going to teach you, has never failed to help those people. It may sound silly and initially you might think how can any one do it and will it work? But precisely by the simplicity of the idea it neutralises the affect of that terrible wrongdoing, which you know is the cause of the persistence of anger/hatred. By the nature of how the human brain works and the default psychological setup, the procedure, which I am going to teach you, will condition you ever so quickly and as a result you will not to be affected by the memory of those wrong doings. Whence you are conditioned which will happen right now, not only will you stop feeling angry/hatred, but also you may be able think about it and talk about it as if it is dead historical memory. Most importantly you have no need to forgive or take any more actions to achieve it."

"So, are you ready? Just focus on the person who caused all this trouble. Make an image of him or her and say it in your mind that he or she will win a lottery or come into a lot of money. He or she will be able to retire and go far away to live in extreme luxury. You may think what justification is there to wish good luck to come to someone who had done something terribly wrong. But you must know that you are only making this statement only in your mind. You have no need to say to his or her face and you know that by simply wishing in your mind will not bring any good luck in reality. The psychological dynamics is that every time the bad memory appears in your thoughts, you simply make a statement in your mind that he or she will come to a good fortune and he or she will retire and go far away to live in extreme luxury. You have to make the statement in full and most importantly you have to do it before any negative emotion, such as anger or hatred settle in your thoughts. Right now, I would suggest that you just think about that person and make that statement."

In almost all the cases the bereaved will laugh with a usual comment " this is ridiculous". KKA will say to the bereaved, "Did you notice that you laughed or you had a smile on your face. The secret of how it works is that when you slap on a positive emotion with good feelings over a memory associated with negative emotion, the negative emotion will neutralise. After repeating a few times without missing any occasion when the negative emotion surfaces, by the processes called conditioning you will find you no longer experience anger or hatred in the slightest. It means that, at last you will stop having the need to endure and suffer from getting angry and hateful. I can assure you that you will soon find yourself having more energy and recover most of your ability to function in full swing and to enjoy the life itself. I want you to keep repeating the statement *right now* until you no longer get angry or hateful." Invariably after three or four minutes the bereaved would express that they are not bothered with that person or what he or she had done. It is not worth feeling angry or hateful any more and they just smile. At this stage of the therapy the bereaved is ready for the final stage of the treatment.

f) **THE FIFTH AND FINAL STAGE** - *Making up all the shortcomings with the deceased while he or she was alive. Simultaneously removing all the negative feelings associated with the last illness of the loved one and the death itself leading to saying "goodbye to the deceased", and finally enriching the life of the bereaved with the treasure of love.*

The time taken to reach the fifth stage would be between three-quarter to one hour in the very first session. The bereaved had been listening to many discussions and was actively involved in neutralizing all the residual negative emotions. It would have involved quoting philosophical metaphors, again using metaphors or in simple language giving scientific clarifications, frank analysis of right and wrong as well as detailed sociological explanations such as commonly held beliefs. Every discussion would be in response to the free, informal and uninhibited expressions of the events or deeds, which had evoked the raw feelings or the negative emotions, which is the whole cause of the harm in the grieving process. KKA would accept the outpouring of every expression wholesomely, non-judgmentally and unbiased.

KKA would sum up everything, which had been dealt with and the outcomes of every issues, just to make sure that nothing had been overlooked or misunderstood. Even if all issues were made good and clear, KKA would remind them of the metaphor of life and the prefixed time for death. He also would underpin the philosophical truth that when the time-to-die is called upon, something had to happen to lead to the death of a person. The death may apparently have been caused by a freak accident like driving a truck straight through a bus shelter or shooting wantonly, or by a deliberate act of violence.

KKA would go over once again before proceeding with stage five to make sure that the bereaved is absolutely sure that all the issues have received satisfactory positive outcome and he or she is certain that not a single issue is left unanswered and no longer carry any guilt, anger or hatred in any form what so ever towards anyone, including him or herself.

Most of the questions raised during the treatment were about pure medical or technical information, which the bereaved wanted to clarify at the time of the death, but did not have time to find out or simply were not offered by the professionals. Sometimes

they felt that they should not trouble the professionals for answers because they took it for granted that they were very busy or beyond their approach. Not uncommonly they were told all the details, but either the bereaved could not remember due the pressure of sadness or they might have misunderstood what they were informed. If the therapist is non-medical and does not know the accurate explanations, then the session has to be terminated and the best thing would be to recall the patient within a week to provide accurate information to the patient. It will give time for the therapist to find the detailed information from the medical colleagues.

Any attempt to skip the part of finding answers or explanations in full to all the questions and no question is too little or insignificant and to proceed with the rest of the package this programme will not work. If the bereaved has not received every answer, which the bereaved is in need of knowing and every single issue is not neutralised, the patient will not be able to *say goodbye to the dead person.* In almost all the cases of therapy for harmful grief, one of the most wanted acts is the saying goodbye. In many cases the bereaved persons had failed to say goodbye to their total satisfaction at the death scene. Therefore in the fifth stage the bereaved is helped to say goodbye to the deceased and fulfil that absolute necessity. The key factor for the total effectiveness in removing the harmful grief permanently in the "Question and Answer Model" is that every bereaved person will have the opportunity to say the proper goodbye and to put a full stop to his or her suffering and it does not matter how long he or she has been suffering. The case histories at the end of this chapter will throw some light on how KKA neutralises anger and guilt or how he makes the answers and interpretations sufficiently effective to make the patient contended beyond doubt. Then only they will be able to say goodbye freely which has to come out of their heart.

*For descriptive purpose, it is simpler to use names for example, in the following description the bereaved is called **Peter** and he is suffering from harmful grief following the death of his father, **John**. Therefore any pretend conversation between John and Peter, each will address to the other as '**father**' or '**son**'.*

At this level of the treatment the bereaved will be very relaxed, contended and peaceful. They are extremely suggestible and highly motivated. They are seeking a way out of the seemingly impassable state of life, which was sad, dysfunctional and twisted around their grief. The experience was almost like being blindfolded and left in a dark forest.

KKA will continue, "What we are going to do now will set you free to become that person you wish to be, without any restriction or reservation. When we finish this session of therapy, you will no longer feel that you are missing the presence of John, your father offering you comfort, consolation and guidance. The most important fact or reality is to understand and firmly believe in, that we have completely removed all the harmful effects of your grief by neutralising all the negative emotions connected with the loss of your love one, your father. Therefore you are now ready to consolidate the realities and you may want to firmly install all those newly acquired understandings as the true facts. This new knowledge of reality is there to stay for the rest of your life as the essential part of your memory, thoughts and feelings in your everyday life. They will remain as the key factor modulating your every interaction with the rest of the world and in turn they will model your reactions and response to everything happening around you. In practical terms, you will start to enjoy having full energy, interest in everything and will regain your full capability and personality you always had. You will spontaneously begin to enjoy being the very kind of person you always wanted to be. You will soon be able to look forward to having a healthy and happy future, which you really deserve. Before we do this part, I must ask you once more, please take a little time to search for any issue or question, anything at all, which are not satisfactorily dealt with. If you find any, however trivial or irrelevant it may seems to you, please bring it out and let us discuss it. If there is one little issue remaining untouched, this programme will not work to the full extent." KKA wait for answer and usually it will be, '**no**'.

Only after getting an absolute 'NO' KKA will continue with the rest of therapy. If necessary, he will persevere with the clearing of any doubts or minor issues, before he will make any progress toward the final part. KKA has found that it is not unusual, the bereaved would only give out minor issues at the beginning, until they become confident and trusting in the therapist, before they would expose the important issue, which might be the cause of the strongest negative emotions.

When both the bereaved and KKA are fully satisfied in clearing all the negative issues, KKA will proceed to set the final but the most powerful and beneficial part of the whole therapy package and that is to help the bereaved to go through the act of "goodbye".

"OK Peter, I want you to sit back. May I have your dominant hand (in this example, right hand)?"

KKA then, lifts the dominant hand to a horizontal position with the palm facing upwards and elbow bent at a right angle and resting on the arm of the chair or on the right thigh. It is important to let the hand rest comfortably, because Peter will be holding it up for a few minutes.

"Peter, I want you to hold the hand as still as you can and keep looking at it. Whatever thoughts might pass through your mind, you must follow what I am going to say. Most importantly do not take your eyes off your hand until I say to do so. If tears flow down, let it run down and do not make any attempt to wipe it or stop it. We will have plenty of time to do that later. Tears are beautiful and have special meaning. If any one has the right to laugh, it is perfectly all right to cry. I would like to assure you of one thing, that I will be with you all the time helping you and giving you all the strength you need to finish what we are going to do. What we are going to do is the most important thing, perhaps in your life, that you would wish to do. I do not want to elaborate or explain any further, because any attempt to describe is the same as doing it."

Looking at the upturned palm, KKA would continue. "Peter, I want you to create a complete image of your father, but do not include any image during the period of his last illness. I repeat, do not include any of the happening during the last illness and certainly any part of the death scene. On the other hand you will have to include everything else, which you remember about your father. I mean, not only just the good times that you had with him, but also the bad times like arguments and fall-outs as well. Then only you will make a complete image and it must be a complete image representing the "whole' of your father, so that you do full justice to him. You must take as long as you need, and do not take any short cuts or omissions."

"You could choose different ways of how to make that image. You could make it like a sculpture, or describe everything in words like on a billboard, or just create a feeling that you just know it is there in your mind. Whichever method you might choose and you don't have to tell me what it is, but you must hold the image of your father in your right hand. I want you to make sure that the formation of the image is taking shape and the final image created must be a **complete image** as I have described. Please don't take your eyes off the image. Until I specifically ask you to stop, you must keep looking at it as you are studying it carefully, adding more detail to make it most real."

It is not unusual that Peter would start crying with sad emotions, as he will have to remember the things, which father and son had done together in the past and those things could never happen in future. If necessary and with the permission, the therapist may want to reinforce the promise of support, by holding Peter's free hand, or just gently supporting the upturned hand from below, or a gentle touch on the shoulder. All such moves had to be done exuding with pure compassion and professionalism. Those gestures of support will certainly encourage the patient to have a catharsis of their dammed up sadness. Such out-pouring of hurt will only result in the greatest relief to the bereaved.

KKA continues. "Do not make any attempt to wipe the tears. They are beautiful in honour of your father and let it flow down as freely as they come, and feel proud of it. When you are as satisfied as it can be with the making of the image, let me know by nodding your head."

Then KKA would wait for the nod, which usually might take five minutes or less. "Now I want you to turn your head this way and look at your left hand." At the same time KKA will take the left hand of Peter and let it rest gently in his hand.

"Do not move the right hand in the slightest from that position, **until I ask you to do so**. In a moment you will know what this is all about. I want you to stop thinking about the image for a moment. I would like to remind you that **until I tell you** please do not look at the image in your right hand, however much you might be tempted to have a look."

KKA will gently lift Peter's left hand with the palm turned up to the same level of the right hand. "Let your eyes focus entirely on your left hand now. As you are concentrating on this hand (KKA holding out the left hand), just imagine that you are sitting by the side of your father in his deathbed. Even if you were not there at the time of actual death, I am asking you to pretend, but put all your heart into that pretence, that you are watching the last minutes of your father's life. He is looking at you now. Peter, please simply pretend that he is, and talking to you, in spite of what has happened. Your father is saying that it is time for him to go, since he has reached 'his port', the end of his journey. In other words John is ready to say goodbye to you. He cannot say goodbye to you, unless you say goodbye to him in return. Goodbye is never a goodbye unless it is done by both of you."

"Before you and your father can say goodbye to each other, I want you to spent a little time reflecting everything which had happened during the last illness (or incident) leading to his death, followed by everything that we had talked about. I really want you attach or put together all the events that go through your mind right now with the image of your father, who is very ill and has reached his port and ready to say goodbye for-ever. I must point out to you that right now, your father is also doing the same as you are, pondering about things had happened during the last few months or moments as the case may be and he may have things to explain or tell you." KKA will remain silent for a short time.

"This time the goodbye is very unique and special, because neither of you will meet again. Therefore the act of saying goodbye has to be done properly and I will guide you all the way to do that, properly. Your father has something to give you, which will be the greatest treasure you will ever have. He is looking at you and waiting for you to say everything that you want him to know. It must include anything you wish to explain to him about something you wanted to do in the past, but never happened because of one reason or other. Now you wish that you had done it a long time ago. This very moment, not only he is listening to every word you say, but also he is asking you to talk to him, right now. He has been wait-ing for this precise moment to exchange goodbyes. He cannot wait any longer, since he has already reached his 'port' to leave this world. In a manner of speaking, it is not fair on him to hang on any longer, as he has to go wherever he is going according to yours and his beliefs. Equally, this moment is your unique opportunity to say goodbye in turn. It is important that you do tell him everything, because everything that you will say now is **the treasure**, which he is going to take with him and will keep in his heart forever. You can say, whatever you have to say as loud as you wish or silently in your mind. Peter, it doesn't matter, as long you say everything. I mean everything. Finally you could see him not only very pleased with you, but also very happy and contended, simply because both of you were able to open your hearts unreservedly. Please do not leave anything behind and certainly no misunderstandings."

KKA will then take the roll of the father, John and make the replies on behalf of him. It would be necessary to create a dialogue between John and Peter to achieve the right degree of impact from the act of "saying goodbye", especially where there was an amount of guilt or misunderstanding in terms of expressed love between them. It allows the bereaved and the deceased to express regrets or any wrongdoing and make the apologies to each other. More importantly they will have a chance to let each other know how much they loved each other in spite of all the shortcomings in the past. Indirectly it will help immensely for those bereaved persons, who always felt that the departed had never loved them enough. KKA may make remarks like, "John understands exactly what you are saying. There is no need to apologise (in a scenario of either of them believing that the love between Peter and John had short comings). You are John's dearest son and he loved you very much, even though he could not properly express his love to you. In spite of what happened between you two, your father knew all long deep in his heart that he loved you just as much as you loved him. All along, deep in your heart, you knew that you loved him as much as he loved you. However neither of you have expressed fully your feelings of love before as you have said it now. It is so wonderful for him to hear you saying how much you loved him. Now he can carry your love in his heart as his greatest treasure and he will take it with him where ever he is going, according to your belief and faith. Not only you can keep his love in your heart, but also he is leaving behind the greatest treasure, which you will receive in a moment, just for you to carry with you, every second of your life."

"He has been waiting all this time (duration from the time of death till the time of treatment), unable to leave his port without saying a proper goodbye. By now you and your father have exchanged all that is necessary to say the proper goodbye. All that is left now is to just say it. He is ready now and he is saying goodbye, he has loved you always and he is very proud of you. Now it is your turn to say goodbye to your father and it is all right to repeat saying how much you loved him. You can see his face with a big smile, looking contented and happy."

As mentioned before that the bereaved would become very emotional while making the image of the departed in his/her dominant hand. The same emotional catharsis will continue through the occasion of saying goodbye. It is important to encourage them to express their emotions freely and unrestricted. Allow the tears to run down. It is always worthwhile to remind them that the benefit of this process, however hard it might feel, will be very comforting for the rest of their life. Words of reassurance of support and guidance, so that they will have full strength to go through the process are just as essential during the goodbye session as it is essential during the image creation. If indicated a gentle pressure on their shoulder (only with their permission) might give them that little extra support they might be wanting.

When Peter started saying goodbye, KKA also says goodbye as if John is speaking, and simultaneously lower the left hand as far down as possible, turning the palm upside down, symbolically dropping all the troubles and sadness associated with the death or loss, as well as anything to do with the last illness, because symbolically KKA has attached the image of John in his last illness and suffering, which Peter has created in his left hand. KKA will make the above symbolic procedure to be felt as real as the absolute truth and fact by saying to Peter, "That is right, Peter, as you are turning your hand upside down, you are actually dropping off and letting go for ever, all that suffering and hurt which your father had to endure during his illness. So please say goodbye to those things as well while you will be saying goodbye to your father." It also means that Peter is letting his father go forever. Saying goodbye is one thing but letting him go and never to return will be very hurtful. On the other hand, all the work KKA and Peter had done so far will create a positive certainty that 'his father has to leave and it is all right for Peter to let him go. Because there is no more unfinished business and all the harmful answers were rewritten with harmless meanings, Peter will feel that no longer he has the need to remain 'frozen' in time at the moment of John's death and perpetually seeking for answers. Even though all the gestures are symbolic, the effect is very profound and practically absolute. Quoting the words of many bereaved how they had felt afterwards, they would spontaneously comment from their heart, that they had regained their "complete self" because they were living with a feeling of incompleteness since they had lost their loved ones along with half of themselves as well. Moreover, Peter will have the real emotional experience and contentment of saying a proper goodbye at his father's deathbed, at the very moment he departed.

Invariably the Peter will let out a large sigh of great relief. Immediately KKA will take the right hand, which Peter has been holding all the time with the palm turned up containing the complete image of his father, John. He will place it over the Peter's chest, lovingly, but surely, at the same time saying, "This is the treasure your father had left for you to keep. You can carry it in your boat. No one can touch it, or take it away from you, or do anything at all to it. This treasure will stay with you forever and where ever you go, always in full and intact. You have no cause or need to look back as every thing you need will accompany you, right by your side in your boat. From now on you can row your boat looking ahead and so you are not going to miss any fish (symbolic to achievements and earnings) on the way. You can catch every one of them as you rightly deserve. There is always someone who could do with the surplus fish that you will catch. From now on you have no need to feel divided, leaving one half behind, as there isn't any thing for that half to do. So re-join and be full again. Now you can spend the rest of your life being the person you always wanted to be, being happy and pleased and being wanted and loved by the people who are close to you. At the same time, from now on you will be able to give your love and care unreservedly to all the people important in your life. It is win, win all round. From now on you can be very contented and comforted knowing your father had gone where ever he might be, being very pleased and happy, because now he knows for sure, that you loved him very much at the same time he knows that his love towards you is clearly accepted by you."

KKA never had a single patient **not** agreeing with the above remarks. On the other hand all bereaved who had been helped by KKA through this treatment package would spontaneously get up and give a hearty hand-shake or even a hug for helping them so much within such a short time. They might have been searching for a way out of their hurt and pain for a long time even many years. They could not be thankful enough.

KKA will summarise the session by telling Peter, "You have learned a lot of things in such a short time. You have a lot to absorb. Not only that you will have a lot to think about during the following few days, but also everything touching your life will be changed. You will have to work out and organise everything within this newly learned emotional framework of good feeling." KKA gives another appointment in two or three weeks time for Peter to return and raise any other issue. Most likely, Peter will phone KKA to let him know how much better he is or he may want even boast about all the new things that he has started to do and how much he is enjoying his life. Quoting one patient's comment, which she said on the second visit, "Doctor Aravind, I have never seen the grass so green for a long time".

Grieving more than one death. Grief can remain and influence the life style of people from the time of the death of their loved ones till their own death. In some cases, harmful grief may exist as a combined affect of more than one death. KKA first deals with the grief, which occupies most prominently in their thoughts. The hierarchy of importance can be established easily. The bereaved usually tell KKA which death is more active. To firmly establish the priority, KKA will simply explain that it is most essential to deal first with the most active grief. Active grief means that the process of grieving preoccupies their thoughts and influences their behaviour everyday; as well as creates more pain and health issues.

The Question and Answer Model of KKA works as educational and as a training experience, in addition to regaining the freedom from the harm of grieving process. Often after the first treatment, which teaches the bereaved how to deal with negative feelings, they themselves may solve issues associated with the remaining deaths. However KKA would specifically ask them to go back to him when any further need comes to light and stresses the importance of making sure that they would complete the resolution process.

POST-THERAPY ISSUES

Occasionally, the bereaved who had been doing very well in their life may need help from KKA for some other reasons. Because they have found life enjoyable and worthwhile, they feel that they would further enhance the quality of their life by entering into a new relationship. They are unsure whether it will be all right to love another person because, in their under-standing or belief, loving a new person might be conceived as unfair to the late partner. They also are unsure whether they will be free to dedicate total love to the new person and so to be fair to him or her. This dilemma is generated from the common belief that one person can posses only one love and it can be relocated only by removing it completely from the deceased partner. The philosophy of love quoted at the beginning of this chapter, was made up by KKA simply to explain to one such patient. The therapist may choose the following three metaphors in that situation, which can arise even in cases of harmless grief.

1. The honey pot metaphor

It is not uncommon that people believe that there is only one piece of love in one life and it cannot be shared without dividing that one piece of love. Therefore such a notion makes them feel guilty for taking away part or whole of that love, which they once gave to the deceased. The very rea-son KKA wrote the paragraph at the beginning of this chapter about how we could look at the phenomenon of love. KKA tells his patients that love is like pots of honey. Rather than having just one pot of honey, which we believe to be shared out between all the people we love, actually we have many pots. The love we have for one person can be likened to having one pot of honey filled to the brim exclusively for that person. A separate pot of honey, filled to the brim to the next person and so on. In other words, always there is a separate pot filled with honey to the brim for each and every person, whom we love. Each pot, which we give, is always full to the brim and the honey in that pot never could or would be shared be-tween more than that unique person. The difference may be in the size of the pot or what the pot looks like from outside. Moreover we can have as many pots as there are people whom we want to love, hundreds if needs to be. We can produce many more fresh pots of love, without emptying or refilling any of the pots, which we already have or for that matter throwing any pot away. All we need to do is just to think in terms taking a new pot for every new relationship fill that pot with love to the brim. Most of us know that the love we give to each other, like our children, grandchildren or other family members and friends, is just as full as the love we had given to the deceased. People, who are actually looking for reassurance and moral support to be happy with life can easily understand and accept this philosophy. The people who were helped by KKA had informed him later that they were very relieved to look at love existing in different pots, which made it easy for them to give full and unrestricted love to someone new, without any reservation or guilt about taking away the love they had given to the departed.

2. The bomb blast metaphor

When a very dear person has departed, the surviving person would feel like a megaton bomb had exploded shattering the pot of his or her life into thousands of pieces. The sound of the blast had deafened all the emotions. The normal feeling would be all jumbled up. Given time the living person will start picking their way up, gathering as many pieces as possible, but never all of them. When they start sticking the pieces together to recreate the pot of life, but never anything like the original, they will find the pot is turning into a new shape and colour, having new usage, fresh purpose and filled with hope. Fresh pieces have to be introduced to fill the gaps, to make the pot stronger, fulfilling new purpose, and to become full and useful once again. So it is perfectly right to take a new relationship as one of the new pieces and it will only make life useful and full again while we are continuing with our own journey.

3. The forest fire metaphor

When people have lost someone very close to their heart, it would feel like a forest-fire burning everything into ashes. The trees are no longer visible, nor do they provide shelter or shade to the animals. But the fact remains, that the stump and the roots of the trees escape from being burnt. They will remain alive under the scorched surface. Some day the rain will fall, the ashes will be washed down to the soil, and the trees will start putting out fresh shoots. This time the tree has the freedom to put its branches in any direction it wishes, to catch more sun, giving it a new shape. The new branches would take up new directions, which they could not do before. In the new life it can cover fresh areas likely to provide better shelter and shade for the animals. There is nothing wrong in having new branches, which will only give fresher pastures and continue to be wanted and useful and so being loved.

People would easily embrace the message in these metaphors and looses all the inhibitions in entering into new loving relationships.

POST SCRIPT

The boat metaphor and the book in heaven metaphor may be used to prevent harmful grief before someone dies, when the death is imminent due to serious illnesses like cancer and other terminal disease. The relatives also may be introduced to the model of how grief can turn into causing harm and encourage them to ask questions during the processes of terminal illness. KKA had used these ideas in a few opportune cases with great benefit in the prevention of harmful grief.

The greatest use for those metaphors is when people who are freshly diagnosed with cancer to enlighten them with a new outlook to life and death. The traditional reaction when a person is told that he/she has got cancer, the light in them goes out and in the shroud of darkness they will start counting the days and hours to meet the death, labelling themselves or by others as *"dying persons."*

KKA has the philosophy for such patients that no body can be a *dying person.* The undisputable reality or the naked truth is that the person is fully alive until the death actually happens. In other words, either a person is alive or dead, and never can be or will be both alive and dead. There is no process of dying, because the shift from the living stage to the dead stage happens in a matter of a millisecond. So they are not dead yet, but living, admittedly having very serious problems. As in the book in the heaven metaphor, death happens to the predetermined time for it. We all know patients with more than one cancer continue to live for many years while people die without being ill for one day in their life. So let us stop counting the days and wasting valuable time and emotion. Instead, why don't we look for ways and means to make a life as good as possible for our own sake and for the sake of the persons close to us until we meet our death? To repeat, we cannot die one second before nor we can delay the death by one second, whatever happens. The gloom and doom feelings about the approaching death will usually mitigate as well as the associated fear and depression. The seriously ill person will become active and positive in their outlook. They will start taking everyday as it comes and filling it with joyful and normal activities to their maximum capability, only restricted by their physical weakness.

The most commonly heard comment or advice, usually made with good intention, to comfort or often to cajole the bereaved could have the opposite effect. Suggestions and comments from well wishers such as, your husband (father, mother, wife or the one who is departed) would want "you to be happy", "you to do this or do that", "it is time you started enjoying your life", "did not want you to be grieving for ever", "get on with your life", "get married again", "go on big holiday or go on a cruise" and so on. Unfortunately such comments are extremely counter productive, because it will only remind the bereaved of the loss of their loved ones. They will feel obliged to carry out something they never wished to do, because they are presented to them as the wishes of the deceased. Any failure will be perceived as disrespectful or unloving toward the deceased because that is "what the deceased would want them do". The bereaved will get into a state of feeling additional guilt on top of the already existing negative emotions, which they are harbouring and causing suffering. More over, because the comments come from persons who are important in their life, such as well wishers, relatives or agents of their faith or professional carers, and because their self-esteem and confidence will be at the lowest level, the bereaved will accept such statements as the righteous and the absolute reality.

Therefore KKA portrays the same motive of giving strength and encouragement to the bereaved to enable them to stand-alone and to make future decisions and engagements for their own happiness, in a very different medium. In situations where the deceased happened to be the dominant person for example a father and son in the relationship, the bereaved may have been highly dependent on the deceased. The bereaved will automatically assume helplessness, requiring continuing approval and skilful guidance from the one who has left them. This is something that they used to enjoy until the time of death. KKA uses the idea of genealogy as a metaphor to fulfil their need. The DNA holds the genes, which make a person who they are and contains the imprints of many skills. The genes are transferred from one person to his or her offspring from one generation to the other, handed down for millions of years. Therefore we all live with an illusion that only our parents have the skills and knowledge to guide us through all situations. This is because we had them as we were growing up and we never gave a thought that we needed to take control ourselves. When they died we believed that we had become helpless without their presence. The fact is that all the skills the parents had were by virtue of the imprints, which they held in their genes. The exact replicas of the very genes are passed on to us and all we need do is to activate them to make us just as skilful as our parents were. The process of activation is simple that all we need to do is simply set upon doing whatever our needs are. Projecting the above notion into the realisation of the "helpless bereaved" will make them acknowledge that they already possess the necessary skills to manage themselves, with out the need to have the presence of their father or mother, who has just passed away. In addition to the above enlightenment, the bereaved will also feel that they are carrying the presence of the departed, because they are carrying the genes of the departed, the basic building blocks of their loved one, which also make them feel that they still have their presence with them as a guide.

Suggested further reading

"Handbook of Bereavement, Theory, Research, and Intervention", *Ed: Margaret S Strobe, Wolfgang Strobe, Robert O. Hansson,* Cambridge University Press, 1993.

"The Path Through Grief", *Marguerite Bouvard with Evelyn Gladu,* Prometheus Books, New York, 1998.

" Healing Grief, A Guide To Loss And Recovery", *Barbara Ward,* Vermilion, London, 1993.

" On Grief and Grieving" *Elisabeth Kubler-Ross and David Kessler,* Simon & Schuster, London2005.

"Bereavement – Studies of Grief in Adult Life", *Colin Murray Parkes,* Penguin Books, London, 1996.

"Gone Forever", Helping children and young people to understand and cope with bereavement and loss. PAVIC Publications, Sheffield Hallam University 1995.

"Sad Isn't Bad" A good grief book for kids dealing with loss (a picture book), *Michaelene Mundy,* One Caring Place, Abbey Press, St. Meinrad, Indiana, 1998.

"The Long Pale Corridor", Contemporary Poems of Bereavement, *Ed: Judi Bensen & Ageneta Falk,* Bloodaxe Books, London, 1993.

"Through Grief", the bereavement journey, *Elisabeth Collick,* Darton, Longman and Todd, London, 1986.

"A Grief Observed" *C. S. Lewis,* HarperSanfrancisco, Harper Collins, 1996.

"The Dynamics of Grief", *David K. Switzer,* Abingdon Press, New York. 1970.

"Bereavement, Studies of Grief in Adult Life New ED", *C M Parkes*, Penguin Books, London, 1998.

Chapter Three

Case Histories

CASE NO: 1

Twenty years ago, this case germinated the seed that prompted KKA to search for the right path of understanding of how grief can harm, and later developed into his "Question and Answer model" in the treatment of grief.

A lady Mrs F, in her fifties approached KKA for intractable facial pains. Her illness started about two and a half years prior to that consultation. She developed intolerance to wearing dentures in spite of the local college of dentistry making different dentures and attempted modifications in each of them over a period of two years. The intolerance to keep the dentures in her mouth progressed to having pain in one side and then spread to both sides of her face. The pain became very disabling in many ways. She had the benefit of neurological investigations and various trials to help her with medications. Because all the investigations had failed to explain the causation of her intolerance and later the suffering of continuous facial pain, as well as all the attempts to invent a suitable denture, she was finally told that nothing more the medical and dental establishments could do for her. Mrs F approached KKA to learn selfhypnosis to control the pain. She knew in her conviction that she was suffering from psychosomatic pain. Traditional self-hypnotic techniques to numb the pain did not help her. KKA had not developed his special grief treatment yet. He set up hypnoanalysis to explore the reason for the failure to self-hypnosis in spite of her having scored highly on the hypnotisability scale.

She recalled the death scene of her husband, which had happened about six months prior the start of her symptoms. It happened on one night, when she went to the kitchen to get a glass of water for her husband. Returning within two minutes, she found her husband dead on the floor and his dentures out on the carpet staring at her. She was shocked. Mrs F revealed that grieving for her husband never entered in her thoughts, because it was not in fashion to think or talk about it. She expected that it was something to accept as a part of any life.

She then talked about a regular nightmare in which *her eldest son was very angry with her because she moved out of their home very soon after the death of his father.* It was their marital home for the past 30 years and they had never lived anywhere else since they got married. In reality, and contrary to the contents of her dream, her son along with many other people were instrumental in recommending her to move out, because all of them believed that it would help her to overcome her sadness and grieving. Mrs F also felt that living in the marital home would keep reminding of their life together and it might aggravate her feeling of loss and sadness. At that point of conversation she began literally wailing and saying how could she do such an injustice to her husband and especially to the beautiful love they cherished between them while they lived in that 'home' for all those thirty years? In her perception, moving out of the marital home was ditching that love. She could not think of any insult worse than her ditching the love of her life and so insulting her late husband. In her words, the shame and guilt caused by her doing that was an "unforgivable crime" and certainly "unpardonable"! Secondly, She felt guilty for not standing up for her wish, which was to continue to live in the marital house. Instead she gave way to her family at the time of intense grief, because she thought what they were saying probably was the right thing to do. Thirdly she blamed herself for leaving her husband by going to the kitchen. If she had stayed, she would know that her husband was in serious trouble and she could have called an ambulance and saved his life. *It shows when someone is suffering from intense grief immediately after the loss of a loved person, how vulnerable he or she would be and how easy it is to solve all the questions by taking the blame oneself.*

KKA neutralised the third guilt by explaining how sudden the death can happen from heart attack without any warning signs to the patient themselves. When she was made aware that she was not a clairvoyant to foresee things, that guilt vanished very quickly.

The second guilt was neutralised by explaining how difficult, if not impossible, for any human being when she or he was dropped deep into intense sadness. She or he would become intellectually paralysed, while the same person has to deal with the grief as well. Therefore the only natural and probably the only way to deal with all the other issues is simply to go along with the advice offered by others without any logical analysis or questioning. In such a situation, all of us would be very weak, confused and so we would make *genuine* misjudgements, which were the norm and not the exception.

KKA usually deals with the least important issue first, in other words, in the reverse order of the hierarchy of importance, because in his experience, the last discussion would be remembered best.

The way the main guilt was neutralised by KKA by explaining to Mrs F, that her marital 'home' was in fact a *building* made of bricks and mortar, like any other *house* was built. Her understanding was that 'love' was similar to material objects and so the bricks and mortar were the beholders of their love. KKA pointed out to her that the experience and feelings of love between two persons was held in their hearts and minds, and never was stored in anything else, certainly not in bricks and mortar! In other words, the persons carried their love, wherever they went. It could not be taken out or *deposited* in anything else. Therefore her love towards her husband had never been lost because it was always and would remain within the *walls* of her heart and mind, irrespective of where she was. KKA reinforced his statement by telling her. "I was born and grew up in India, 6000 miles away from the UK. When I came over to live in the UK, I did not leave the precious love, which I held towards my family and friends in India. On the contrary, I carried it with me *deep in my heart* and I could still feel it right here (putting his hand on heart) *untainted and undiminished*. Likewise you always carried your love in your heart and your husband carried his love in his heart and surely he had taken it with him wherever he had gone to." Immediately she remarked, "why wasn't I thinking like that?" She recognised how the metaphors reflected the truth. Mrs F looked a little foolish, but greatly unburdened. KKA went on telling her that, "when you are faced with too many hurtful things and when you are incapable of dealing with them, you have to set some of them, if not most of them, aside and make an effort to move on in life. There is always a specific time for everything to happen and in your life the time for putting things in their true perspectives happened to be right now, when we are having this discussion." *The last statement was made to avoid the possible creation of a new guilt or undervaluing her intelligence or capability, because she might start blaming herself for not sorting the issues much earlier by logical thinking and she could have avoided a lot of her suffering, etc. etc.*

Mrs F was miraculously cured of her pains and she could tolerate any kind of dentures! KKA saw her only ten years later with gallstones, as she remained in good health. She had lived a very active and contented life.

CASE NO: 2
This case illustrates how grief can turn harmful from simple and innocent misunderstanding.

One female patient 'Mrs CF' in her late forties was attending the surgery of KKA with multiple complaints over a period of three years. All her illnesses presented as pains in one organ at a time. When the first one was treated, the pain reappeared in another organ. Having a few surgical and medical interventions in the course of treating her fleeting pains, she began to experience severe anxiety. She became disabled because the anxiety compounded with the pains. She could no longer hold on to her job. Grave fear of heading for serious physical illness and her own recognition of herself as 'a wreck' caused great family upset and breakdown of household harmony. She was genuine about her suffering. Mrs CF used to be a healthy and very family orientated person.

All her ill health started about a month after the death of her father, who was under the care of KKA. KKA had introduced his grief prevention to the whole family. The mother of Mrs CF was able to have a normal harmless grief and a fairly normal life. However, when Mrs CF asked for help to manage her anxiety KKA doubted the possibility of grief being a factor. Until then she had never talked about her father or her grief over his death, even though she had seen KKA many a time for the pains, which she was having in various organs. Suspecting grief might be a contributing factor to her sufferings, KKA decided to expose her to the memory her father, indirectly by asking how her widowed mother was coping and living alone since her father' death? Mrs CF appeared rather abrupt, in a stern voice she said that her mother was doing all right, 'rather too well'. Then Mrs CF began to cry. During further conversation she expressed her fear that she would never get out of her current predicaments because she did not deserve to be happy in life. In other words, she was guilty of the terrible thing that she had done. So she must be a very bad person. KKA then asked her directly, whether she was grieving for her father? She could not hold her tears.

She was brought back for proper grief treatment as described. She was carrying a huge amount of guilt. She really wanted her father to be cremated. She should never have agreed to her mother's wish of burying her dad. She could not bear the thoughts of her dad being eaten away by hundreds of worms, in his grave. She should have insisted otherwise and so it was her fault that her father was left in the soil to be eaten away by worms. On serious discussion, she remembered some horror movie in which how all-dead bodies had disappeared in the coffins, instead they were full of nasty worms. KKA explained to her how dead bodies degenerate inside coffins, by the action of tiny bacteria and chemicals released from the body itself, like what she might have seen in fruits degenerating (KKA deliberately avoided the word "rotting") in storage. More over KKA told her that he had seen coffins intact when exhumed years after burial. She loved her mother just as much she loved her father and so her mother had equal rights if not more in making the decision to cremate. Mrs CF remarked that a great load had gone from her, which was expressed in physical terms by straightening herself from a crumpling posture. She was able to say goodbye to her father during the final package of grief treatment by KKA. During the goodbye she apologised for having the misunderstanding and how much she loved him. From that moment on Mrs CF returned to her good health and back to work and regained the family happiness.

CASE NO: 3
This case shows how harmful grief can masquerade in the form of serious illness

Female patient H of 50 years of age sought help from KKA. Out of the blue, H collapsed and she could not walk or even stand up. Thorough neurological examination and extensive investigations as an inpatient, failed to explain her problem. She needed physical help to go to the toilet and even for getting dressed. That state of disability went on for six months, in spite of psychiatric treatment and antidepressants. She entered the consulting room of KKA holding onto, and supported by, her husband. Both of them accepted that there must be a psychological basis to her suffering.

Discussions revealed she had a lot of guilt and anger connected with her late husband. The anger was towards the family of her husband, who were very vindictive towards her and even hid the details from her, where her husband was buried stopping her from visiting his grave. She was ostracised from her husband's family, soon after his death. Her anger was fully justified to have and it was not out of distorted perception.

KKA used what he calls as "the 3 option strategy" as previously described. In the case of Mrs H the third option helped her to get rid of all the anger.

Once the anger towards her ex-in laws had neutralised, Mrs H revealed a mountain of guilt. The guilt only showed up when she remarried and began to enjoy the new love and life. She realised that she could be very relaxed and enjoy an uninhibited sexual relationship in her new partnership. Due to some reason, completely unknown to her, she had had great difficulty in having a relaxing union with her late husband, even though she truly loved him. Mrs H began to question in her own mind why she had behaved badly towards her first love, denying him many things she felt should have done and could have given many happy moments. On the other hand, whilst she spent life with her first husband, she did not think that there was anything wrong in her behaviour and she was so naïve to take it for granted that was quite normal in a marriage. She turned much wiser only after she had met her second husband. Her guilt was immense filled with regrets, all founded over the things she denied from her first husband. Only when she talked about the guilt she realised that she was grieving for him. Until then she was preoccupied with the anger towards her in laws.

This case shows suppressed harmful grief can lie hidden until something to trigger it at a later stage. One could assume that her anger towards the family of her late husband was strong enough to dissociate the grief from her awareness and so it remained suppressed.

The guilt began to appear about a year after the re-marriage. It reached a crescendo, when she decided to dispose of articles belonging to her first husband. KKA was able to bring out her hidden fear of having children, from an incident as a teenager witnessing her aunt having a highly traumatic and life-threatening childbirth. That psychological trauma was the inhibiting factor in her behaviour towards her late husband by denying him children. KKA pointed out to her that, she could not be blamed for her behaviour because as far as she was concerned, getting pregnant equated to death. The fear was so strong she had even blocked out the memory of witnessing, in her own word, the "horrendous" experience, as she had perceived the traumatic childbirth. KKA gave her relevant explanation to alter he perception and successfully removed the fear. She had entered into the menopause by the time she married again and the underlying psychological anxiety became irrelevant, as she would not get pregnant. Mrs H understood the unconscious reasoning for her very opposite behaviours with the late husband and the present husband. She could readily accept that there was no reason for her to feel guilty any more on any of her behaviours, past or present. She could also accept that she had the right to enjoy future life, to love and be loved. Within the framework of KKA's grief therapy she was able to explain the reason for her actions and say a proper goodbye to her late husband. Within weeks after the treatment she started to drive and got out of all her symptoms. KKA had followed her for over10 years and she remained problem free.

CASE NO: 4
This case has an unusual presentation of symptoms affecting her personal and family life when she started to grieve over her own <u>assumed death</u>.

A young married woman, KT, in her twenties was enjoying good health and a loving relationship. When her only son reached three years of age, she suddenly started suffering from anxiety, fear of the unknown, depression and loss of libido. She was distraught, but she could not reason out the underlying cause. When questioned about what passed through her mind, whenever she thought about her condition, especially when she was describing her symptoms to KKA. She said that an image of her son being without his mother kept appearing in her thoughts all the time. She was very disturbed even when she had to say it out loud. This was quite understandable when the image was clearly indicating that she would be dead soon to make her son motherless. When KKA asked her to describe that cryptic statement in a different way, she started crying. She stated to KKA that she would die like her mother, who died when she was only nine years of age. KT had not uttered a word about those thoughts to anyone else and carried on suffering in silence. She carried the feeling of great loss and the sadness being denied of the normal pleasures and love, which her friends enjoyed having a mother and the things a daughter and mother would have done. KT mentioned that she could not recall any specific event, which triggered the present feelings. Almost straight away she said with surprise that, she was experiencing grief for her mother, who had died nearly sixteen years ago. KT had no memory of grieving for her mother until that day having the consultation with KKA. No one else she knew had fallen ill to indicate an impending death. The only factor that she could think of, which might have any connection with her current state was her son is growing up and soon he would reach the age, when she had lost her mother. Whatever might have triggered the grief, KKA offered her to give the full treatment of grief, which she readily agreed to have.

Talking about the circumstances surrounding the death of her mother was that her mother had been admitted to a hospital with an acute illness of some sort and she never saw her mother again. Nobody told the nine-year-old child what had really happened, apart from saying that her mother had gone to heaven. KT wanted to see her mother very badly but the adults would not allow her to see her dead mother, giving no explanation as to why she was not allowed. KT was not taken to the funeral. She missed her mother badly and very importantly the fact of saying goodbye when her mother departed for her journey to heaven. All she received from the grown-ups was a stonewall silence or they would tell her to be quiet when she raised any questions. KT's main issue was that she did not have a chance to say goodbye to her mother. Great regret that she could not attend the funeral clouded her feelings all the time as she was growing up. The mystery to her and to KKA was that the nature of her feelings as she was growing up she did not accept as sadness; but automatically accepted the way she felt was normal to anyone without a mother. It had never occurred to her that there was a need to do anything about it. The reality of the rawness of her suffering only revealed itself during the consultation with KKA.

KT received full grief treatment from KKA within the same session of consultation. All the metaphors with special emphasis on the 3-option-strategy were used to explain the behaviour of the elders during the last illness and the funeral of her mother. She was able to say goodbye to her mother and tell her how much she loved her and how much she had missed her. The effect of the treatment was immediately apparent. When she was reviewed two weeks later, she was feeling good and had started enjoying sex again, to the relief of her loving and dedicated husband. She noticed positive changes in her son, seeing her happy and relaxed. KKA followed her up for few more years until he retired from practice and all the while KT remained well.

CASE NO: 5
This case is rare, because the grief began to affect her from childhood. She was grieving the loss of her twin brother, who was still born. The treatment of her grief by KKA was spread out during a period of nearly 20 years. It went through most of the evolutionary stages of KKA's "Question and Answer Package"

MD in her late fifties came to the attention of KKA during a routine consultation in his daily practice. She presented with depression, which she described, as "everything is very dark". She could not do her work, for that matter, anything. Apart from holding a high level job, she was about to receive a high academic accolade. MD wanted to throw away all her hard work, because she could not think of any achievement, which she was worthy of. The depression was treated with medication along with analytical interviews to explore her underlying thoughts. She came up with having a great deal of guilt. Most of the guilt was generated from impositions from her family. She was one of the twins who her mother was carrying in her first and only pregnancy. The other twin, a boy, did not survive the childbirth. The confinement was very complicated and all her life she was reminded by both of her parents, especially by her mother, that her birth nearly killed her mother. Her mother never got pregnant again. MD was made to believe that she was to be blamed for putting her mother's life in danger as well as causing the stillbirth of her twin brother. MD also took the blame on herself for delaying the delivery of her twin brother by coming out first and she strongly believed that the delaying caused her twin brothers' life. As she began to get older, MD genuinely passed the sentence of great guilt onto herself and started grieving for her twin brother. The presenting crisis was triggered by the possibility of receiving the academic accolade.

All the misconceptions regarding the death of MD's brother were removed with medical explanations and the guilt associated with the death was neutralized. Until she received the treatment MD resented her parents often reminding her of the difficult birth and the loss of their son. Her perception was that they cared and loved the son they never had more than they loved her. KKA was using hypnosis and other metaphor to help her with her guilt and related misconceptions about how she perceived her parents thought about her. She remarked that how strange it was to construe one's own understanding, when she realised by herself that the frequent mentioning by her parents all through MD's life of her late brother was only because they were also grieving. Most importantly she acknowledged that the strength of guilt and grief made her believe that her parents did not care or love her and how wrong it was to have such a notion. Being highly intelligent MD herself was able to explain the dynamics of such twisted misconception, that a guilt in her made her create the notion of her unworthiness and also might be the reason for her perception of her parents not loving her as much she wanted, but in reality, they did love her and cared for her very much. However, when the guilt and grief had seemingly resolved she could clearly accept the reality of how much they actually loved, cared and valued her, simply because they did encourage her to go to university and they did fully support her through every bit of her career, especially because they came from a working class society and were not rich. She made a remarkable recovery and secured her academic accolade. However MD needed help and support now and then for the next twenty years, for relapses of anxiety and depression, certainly in a minor degree.

While leading an active life, at the age of eighty, MD started getting upset and depressed again. She then told KKA that, she was missing her brother and that her guilt of leaving her brother to die resurfaced. The fact remained that MD had not managed to say goodbye to her twin brother. When KKA helped MD about twenty-five years ago, he had not developed the model fully to include helping to say goodbye. On that occasion, KKA helped her to say a proper goodbye. At the end of the therapy, she told KKA that she was able make her brother understand the medical issues behind his non-survival, which he could accept and in fact she confabulated an image of her helping him rather than leaving him to die and both of them hugged each other before parting. The great relief on her face was astonishing and eventual happiness and contentment prevailed during the rest of her life.

CASE NO: 6

This case was interesting because the grief treatment was carried out by letters between KKA in UK and the aggrieved family who lived in Kerala, India. The family had held great respect for KKA and it helped towards the success of process. While working as a general surgeon in Kerala, Mr R received treatment from KKA when Mr R was admitted with multiple fractures of the skull and tear of the sagittal sinus. KKA managed to repair the damage achieving full recovery. Soon after KKA returned to UK.

Twenty years later, Mr R died suddenly of meningitis. Until then he was enjoying excellent health. A common friend informed KKA by letter, the sad tragedy and how much the widow and the grown up children were suffering from grief. KKA responded with a letter addressed to the son of Mr R, as cited below with the permission of the family.

"With great sorrow I came to know through our common friend Dr N, the saddest news of the untimely demise of Mr R. I was much shocked. It took me many days thinking about the kind of letter I could write to you. I sincerely apologise for the time it took in sending this letter. I would not be able even think of the depth of your grief and sadness.

I vividly remember that your father, mother and you with your two sisters sat down for a sumptuous meal, when my wife and I came to your house about seven years ago. It seems as though it was yesterday. I thought then "what a lovely family you were". We were fortunate to see your father again in February this year, as he dropped in at the hotel where we were staying. We really regretted that we could not meet you, your mother and sisters, because that trip to Kerala was a short visit.

As you know, my first encounter of R was in 1973, when he was laid on the operating table in the hospital in Kerala, where I was working as the surgeon. He was unconscious after sustaining one of the most serious head injuries, literarily smashed up skull. I operated on him patching the torn up vein in the brain and wired up all the pieces together. With his courage and determination he made complete recovery to normality. My memory of him remains very clear in every detail. My first impression of him was "what a strong person he is" while he was recovering from that injury. The more I came to know him, the more I grew very fond of him with great admiration and respect for the kind of a person he was. Especially, whenever I thought of him, one thing that always came to the front my memory was his laughter, so natural, exuding with kindness and friendliness. He was a generous and friendly man.

After all these years in medical practice and being a part of many people's lives from the beginning to the end, I have grown to become a firm believer in what many people call 'The Fate' or what I would like to call the '**Inevitable**'. There are two '**Inevitables**' in everyone's lives. One inevitable is the **time** when we start our life and the other is the **time** when we meet the end of it. Those two times are prefixed even before we start the journey of our life. Those two times are not negotiable, meaning they have to happen whatever the circumstances are. Nothing, not even God, can change or shift either of them. We are **living** from the very first moment when we start our life and likewise we are **living** until the very last moment to the end our life. Between those times we will have to be doing something or something will happen to us. Therefore, whatever happens to us just before our death is not the real cause of our death. However we always attribute the cause of death due to whatever had happened or whatever that we had done leading to the moment of our death. The actual reason for the **precise moment** when we die is always that we have reached our **prefixed time** and **not because** of something has happened to us at the time of our death. In other words, it is our '**Inevitable**' makes something happen and it could be any one of the many things. We would label anyone of the happenings as the one, which killed or caused the death. The following storey may be helpful to understand what I believe, which I do very strongly, in spite of my ardent scientific background. It has helped many people including myself.

KKA quoted the "Book in Heaven" metaphor in full in this space of the letter.

We all have to die when it is our time to die and not one moment early or one moment late. It makes no difference in whatever we are engaged in or whether we are well or ill. Even if we are very ill and if the time to die has not reached, in spite of everything we have to keep on going until we reach that time. On the other hand when the time is right, something has to happen and something will happen, which will be labelled as the cause of death. Gripped with intense sadness, as a natural human response, the bereaved would constantly look back at such things labelled as the cause of death laden with questions whether something different could have happened or done, which might have saved his life. The answers, which you could accept, had to be something that would have saved him from death and so he might be still alive. We hear such comments almost all the time after someone's death, like in the famous story of Julius Caesar, who would not have been stabbed to death, if he had listened to his wife's heart breaking plea to him not to go out that night. We always ask such questions whenever death or tragedies happen. No death or partings ever escape from such questioning at least by someone, if not most of us. What had happened had happened, but it would only happen if the time were right. So please do not think that something would have saved Mr R. In the same way, please do not ask "why him" and "why on that day". R had always said that he could have died when he received the terrible head injury, if not for KKA who gave him a second life. He always insisted that he was reborn with full faculties. I am sure that all of you have heard him say that many a time. However, R catching meningitis was simply that the right time for him to leave this world had come and it wasn't to be a moment before or a moment after.

Let us value his time that he had on this earth. Let us think of all the things that we can remember of him, including all good things and equally all the bad things; the things which we disagreed with him; the times when he might have made us angry or whatever. But please do not include the details of his last illness, because that belongs to the *goodbye* time. Let us make a **total** image of him with all the good and all the bad things in it. Let us look at it as the most valuable treasure that he had left for us, which each and every one of us can keep in our own heart **forever**. We can take it with us wherever we go, until it is our time to say *goodbye* to the others and leave this world. Just let us imagine, putting all our heart into that imagination that we are there by his bedside, just at the time he has reached the end of his journey.

"Let us say to him how much **we loved**, how much **we thought of him.** Tell him that our true love, which he will be taking from us to carry in **his heart** wherever he is going after his departure from this world. With a big smile on his face he is saying to us how much he loved us and thought of us and how much he put his family first, all the time. It is time for him to say **goodbye** to us and us to him, because he and us understand that it is time for him to go.

Now he and we have already exchanged treasures, please join in bidding him **goodbye** as he is saying **goodbye** to us, at the same time he is saying goodbye to his last illness too. He is smiling because he has got a treasure from us to take with him and also he now knows that we have the treasure from him to keep in our hearts, miss him any time in our life. **Goodbye.**"

> Please be in touch with me. When I come to Kerala next
> time I will make every effort to meet you. Love to all

> Aravind

KKA received a letter from his son. Apparently, when Mr R was very ill with meningitis and became confused, he was asking when his father, who had died few years ago, was coming to see him as expected. The three children believed that their grandfather was the messenger from God and took their father away. They were very happy with that concept. KKA's letter gave them lot of comfort. Their mother, wife of late R, was very much worried, because she thought that the death of R might be due to some form of carelessness from her side i.e., by not giving proper and enough food to fill his stomach when he was gravely ill with meningitis and that might have weakened him and caused him to die. It made her to feel very guilty and not worth living. The family tried to explain to her that patients cannot take full meals when they are exhausted and seriously ill. She would not accept any of the explanations from her children or from anybody, but stayed with her guilt. However, after reading the letter KKA had sent, she admired that her husband caught meningitis and died because "God has decided likewise". She let her guilt go away as well.

KKA visited the family during his next trip to Kerala and found everyone moving on with their life as normal as they could, though they remained sad that they had lost R, but they did not carry any negative feelings.

CASE NO: 7

KKA had personal experience of grief. That experience added insight into the development of his model, which expresses the high significance of saying proper goodbye. Whatever reasons there might have been, harmful grief may develop if the slightest doubt in the thoughts of the bereaved exists that they were not able to or they did not have the chance to say goodbye properly. That imperfection or missing section will make the grief to remain unresolved, in other words, it will continue being harmful.

KKA just entered into general practice in England. He was struggling with finance to pay the mortgage, car hire and supporting the family. In 1976 his father, who lived in India, died after a short illness. KKA did not have the money to make his journey for the funeral. KKA tried to get a bank loan and was turned down. It took three years before KKA could visit his hometown in Kerala. Mr V was the closest friend his father had, though Mr V was three years older than him. Mr V had held very high regards and affection towards KKA. MR V was present in the room when KKA's father died.

KKA called in to see Mr V. KKA saw him laid in bed looking much older and frail. Mr V in a very weak voice expressed the pleasure of meeting KKA. He revealed that he missed his close friend and he thinks about him almost everyday. His eyes were filling with tears and the sadness was obvious. Mr V was clearly grieving the death of KKA's father. KKA sat down on the bed both facing each other. KKA realised that he also was grieving. Suddenly, it occurred to him that the unusual tiredness, which he was suffering for the past two years, was connected to his grieving. Being in a busy general practice and bringing up a young family, KKA did not think the possible association of his tiredness and the grief for his father. More to the surprise of KKA, Mr V also was waiting for the presence of KKA to unleash his grief, as if he needed KKA as a witness. KKA was carrying some amount guilt that he could not have made that journey when his father died. He needed to say a proper goodbye to his father, but he did not know how it could be done.

Sitting down on Mr V's bed and facing each other, both began talking spontaneously about the good and the bad, in other words everything, about KKA's father. KKA would tell one thing, which would be taken up by Mr V who would add something more to it or take up another event, like joining pieces of a jigsaw puzzle. Some of the materials, which were commonly known to both, but a lot of them were about experiences, which were known only to one of them. Both were reminiscing many things and laughing at times, but neither took any notice of the flood of tears from their eyes, literarily soaking the clothes and even the bed. They were automatically constructing a true memory of KKA's father.

One of the issues raised was how impossible it was for KKA to get the money to attend the funeral. Mr V highlighted the fact that they did not have the facility to keep the body for more than ten hours before it had to be cremated. In the tropical heat the body decomposes very quickly. Mr V pointed out the simple fact that the funeral would have been done and dusted even before KKA could board the flight from the UK. In other words even if KKA had made the journey from the UK he would not be able to attend the funeral. Moreover Mr V had gone through hard times in his life. He told KKA that he could perfectly understand the problem of not having money. MR V helped KKA to neutralise the guilt, which he was carrying as he believed that he could have attended the funeral if he had had the money. What surprised KKA was that he had never thought of that simple reality, until he had met Mr V three years later. Then of course, KKA knew the explanation for that blind belief. This was simply formed by the strength of his sadness and grief from the loss of his father. From then on KKA stopped feeling guilt. *How the human mind works is that, even though the reality is quite plainly known to KKA especially with his expertise in human psychology, he would remain incapable of accepting it as a valid explanation, which could have neutralised his emotional guilt at any time before, but he had to wait until someone else explained the same reality.*

Neither Mr V nor KKA moved an inch all through their encounter, which lasted for two hours, did they never try to wipe their tears. At the end of the construction of the complete history or the image of the very much loved father to KKA and a very much loved friend to Mr V and when both of them knew that there was nothing more to add, together they said goodbye to KKA's father. They thanked each other. As KKA was about to leave Mr V remarked that he was waiting for KKA to visit him, as he could not bid goodbye to his friend without the presence of KKA and no one else. Mr V and KKA bid goodbye to each other. Both of them felt that they had freed themselves of a great load from their mind, which they were carrying. *That spontaneous, un-trained and unrehearsed behaviour gave KKA the material to shape his programme of saying the final good-bye and it could be done any time after the death.*

CASE NO: 8
This case enlightens the utmost need to say goodbye to the fullest satis-faction, in order to avoid harmful grief and it was not enough being pres-ent at the bedside when the loved one died.

Mr B took ill with multiple myeloma, in his early fifties. During that period KKA was highly involved with using hypnosis in the management of cancer for minimising the side effects of chemo/radio therapy. The hypnosis package involved not only helping to create a high quality of useful life for the patients, but also nurturing a deep understanding amongst the relatives for them to be able to accept the final outcome. KKA was using the grief therapy package as an integral part of his approach.

About two months after the death Mr B, his widow approached KKA for help, because she felt lacking in confidence. She also felt that she did not deserve to be happy. She could not comprehend what was making her feel "being shackled", even though she failed to identify any issue. She had the benefit of KKA's grief therapy package while her husband was alive. KKA used it to prevent the grief becoming harmful.

KKA went through with her all her thoughts and feelings step by step. It revealed that, at his bedside in the hospital, she was with Mr B holding his hand all the time to the very end. She remembered that Mr B was trying to say something like bidding goodbye to her just before he died. But she missed the chance to say goodbye back to him before he became unconscious and died, because she was overwhelmed with sorrow, floods of memories and thoughts of the future, at the same time she had to take care of everything else, such as making him as comfortable as she could. She felt awfully guilty and stupid for not saying how much she loved him. She only needed the last part of KKA's grief package and that was to exchange goodbyes. KKA set up a kind of pretend dream that she was sitting at the bedside at the hospital and asking her to imagine that she was reliving the last moments of Mr B's death scene. She was able to recreate the scene in her imagination giving all her heart into that pretence. Soon she began to experience that everything was really happening as if she were at the death scene. KKA helped her to say a proper goodbye to Mr B as previously mentioned in the grief treatment package to her total contentment. Three months later she came back and told KKA that she took driving lessons and passed the test; she had bought a new car and got a new job and was having a productive life style. She was followed up for many years and remained free of harmful grief.

CASE NO: 9

This case represents how long harmful grief can remain concealed, even though the bereaved never had a single day without the torment from the guilt associated with her son's death.

Mrs C was a highly intelligent health professional. KKA was involved when Mrs C found it too traumatising to attend a training course involving children's health. Half way through the course she decided to give it up. KKA happened to be her personal tutor as well as one of the lecturers. During the discussion to explore the causes for her to feel that way and because she started the course with great enthusiasm and was scoring high levels of marks, he had to ask her whether there could be a possibility of grief playing a part in her feelings,

She told KKA that she struggled to go through each and every day since her nine-year-old son died from cancer about ten years ago. At work and with her family and friends she had to pretend that she was as normal as anybody else, whilst inside the torture of guilt burned relentlessly. She was not able to whisper a single note to anybody about it, until that very moment when KKA asked the question of grief. Being her personal tutor KKA had developed a good rapport with her and so she had no hesitation to talk about her trouble to him.

Her son was admitted to hospital for terminal care. The medical team were not controlling his pain well. The child had told about his pain only to his mother. Mrs C conveyed her concern to the medical team and she was reassured that he was getting all the necessary medications. However he was really suffering from pain. Being connected with health care Mrs C knew there were other effective medications, which could relieve "her little helpless boy from pain". The consultant turned the request down on the basis of the many "serious side effects" of the drug in question. She was unable to question or argue with the consultant, because of her own distress seeing her son suffering. She did not consider demanding to get the drug prescribed, but went along with whatever was being offered. The child had to endure a long period of distress before he died.

A few months after the death, she began to think more critically of anything and everything as grief was hurting her very strongly. Her analysis took her straight into the issue of his pain relief and what she "should" have done to help her son's last journey of life a little more pleasant. It did not take much deliberation before her traumatised mind, deep in sorrow arrived at a judgement and the verdict. *"She should have questioned the consultant and insisted that her son should get stronger medication to free him from pain irrespective of the side effects".* Looking back, he only lived for a couple of weeks in pain. According to her thinking, any side effects would not have mattered at all. The most important issue, as far as she was concerned, should be always the control of his pain at any cost. She could not think of any excuse for her not to demand that her son should be given the most effective drug. She was the mother and she felt that it was entirely her responsibility and duty to help him. She had failed in her parental obligation. All this criticism, analysis and judgements only started after his death. The guilt was enormous and she sat on it, suffering in silence for ten years. *It is very typical how sadness and grief can distort judgements and how the verdicts can become absolute and unquestionable!*

KKA explained to her the absolute truth about the human mind. It could process only one thought at any one moment, which in turn is determined by the emotional happenings at the same time. Because we could only have one thought during a given time, we could only hold one belief during that specific time. As it would be the only belief, opinion or decision in any given moment, that belief would be acted upon as absolutely *the right thing* to do at that moment. No human could do anything else, better or worse, but to act to the letter of that belief. Therefor nobody deserved to be blamed, or made guilty for something that person had done, believing it was the right thing to do to the best of his or her understanding at the time of his or her action. It never was an option to do differently. The understanding would change only later on, when the outcome of that act became available and never before. Again the out come would certainly depend upon many other events taking place, which were absolutely unpredictable. In the case Mrs C, if someone could predict that her son would die soon as it happened, the consultant would have given the medications with serious side effects, on the other hand, it would not be the right choice if he happened to live longer. In a way, the consultant, to his best of judgement, believed at that time that he had taken the right decision. Therefore there was no reason for Mrs C to carry the guilt, as there was no guilt involved. Mrs C would be guilty if she did something against her belief at the time of her original decision, but it would never be possible any way.

KKA brought his favourite 'God Metaphor', as previously described, to support his explanation to change her guilty verdict to a not-guilty verdict. Even God had made mistakes or overlooked things because he was busy, and so how could we, the humble human beings be above God and should expect not to make any mistakes? Making mistakes should not be considered as guilty. We had to learn from our mistakes and use that knowledge in future to understand things differently and if possible not to repeat the same mistake. It was not meant to make one guilty.

Mrs C sat in silence for a while contemplating. A smile of relief and contentment appeared on her face. She was able to feel that there was no need to feel guilty. She was freed from that guilt. The newly found positive feeling required reinforcement then and there to make certain that Mrs C would never question or go back on the newly learned understanding and that was, in no way she was guilty of her allowing the consultant to decide upon the medication. KKA further comforted her by explaining that the processes of finding herself guilty had happened because of her extreme love for her son and the immeasurable hurt following his death. **Under such circumstance we search for something to be blamed to underpin that hurt.**

KKA further neutralised the affect of guilt on her by asking Mrs C to make a conversation in her imagination with the *Mrs C, who was ten years younger* who had started with the guilt feeling. The conversation would have to be giving explanation how the guilty verdict was formed in the first place and how the newly learned wisdom had removed that guilt completely. The older Mrs C, who was in conversation with KKA had to install the reformed, not-guilty verdict in the younger Mrs C and make the younger Mrs C feel completely contented with the change of feeling, in other words, to feel OK about what she had done ten years ago. After a few seconds of silence, the older Mrs C revealed that the ten years younger Mrs C had accepted the explanations in full and as a result both Mrs Cs felt positively sure that they loved their son and did their best as they thought and believed to be the right thing they could ever possibly do. The older Mrs C's face lit up and she couldn't thank KKA enough, for freeing her from the long standing suffering of guilt and the very dysfunctional life during the previous ten years.

Because of the feeling of guilt, she had not said a proper goodbye to her son. Apart from that, she did not have any other issues. KKA took her through the goodbye part of his grief treatment package. During the goodbye she was explaining to her son how it was and what she did was to the best of her knowledge and how much she loved him. She said afterwards, that she could see a smiling and happy face of her son as he said goodbye to her at the same time he reassured her that he always knew that she loved him and had always given him her best. In turn he had always loved her. She continued with the course and secured distinction in the final examination.

CASE NO 10

This case brings certain facts how lack of understanding can cause harmful grief.

Mrs N approached KKA saying, "I want to pick your brain." She wanted to know whether it was all right to take sleeping pills because the antidepressants, which she was prescribed, were not helping her to sleep.

KKA casually enquired, what made her think that she was depressed? She replied that most of her family had said so. Her family and friends alike told her that she was inadequate and nasty towards people who were closer to her. Mrs N interpreted their comments as they all were picking on her for no good reason. She did not know what to do. She began to cry and sob. Between sobs she said that she missed her husband a lot who died about 4 years ago from cancer. She wanted to know why she was feeling so bad and sad. It was four years since her husband died. Surely, one should have got over it by this time. She admitted that she did not like to be alone at home. Apart from the loneliness she had no cause for anxiety.

By this time it became obvious that she was holding on to grief, which was harming her in terms of loss of self-esteem, increased physical tiredness, undervaluing her abilities, overwhelming her with thoughts of unworthiness and she had no right to enjoy life. Mrs N felt that she did not deserve even to ask for help. Those feelings were generating cyclical anxiety and depression.

In the case of Mrs N she had been getting help from KKA for one symptom or other during the previous four years. Every second of her waking life she was well aware of the feeling of guilt associated with her husband's death, but she never suspected grief could be the cause of her problems.

Most often people affected by harmful grief will consult KKA with other mental or physical problems but rarely as grief per se. The issue of grief will only surface much later during the discussion or even after many years of going through different ailments. There are many possible explanations for such behaviour. KKA believes that the main force behind the concealment of grief or being blind to grief is their guilt and the attached negative verdicts loaded with shame and unworthiness. The evidence for that view comes from the statements made by the bereaved after KKA had successfully treated them for grief. They would spontaneously remark at the follow up meeting since the completion of the treatment, that how much their self-esteem has come back and they can hold their head high with pride and satisfaction. In other words, KKA's Question and Answer package not only neutralises the negative verdicts, but also elevate them to the opposite spectrum of positive emotional status.

The other reason for grief not being the presenting symptom is whenever anyone attempts to discuss the issue of grief, the whole bulk of negative emotions peak up and lead them to re-live the moments of death of their loved one. As a result they have to endure another addition of pain and hurt on the top of the existing level pain and hurt. The agony can be hard to bear and often they back off from opening any discussion of their grief.

There always is a time for everything to happen in one's life. Often by chance that day becomes the time in one's life for those issues of grief to be brought into discussion. The intervening time is also determined by chance and so unpredictable. It is worth remembering that when they attend for their first treatment for whatever reasons they will show all the physical expressions indicating deep emotional suffering.

KKA invited Mrs N to undergo grief treatment and assured her that it would help her. For the details of the treatment package, please refer to that chapter. She began to describe what had happened during the last few days of her husband who died of cancer. She started with trivial issues like her husband did not talk about how serious his cancer was.

When KKA explained to her that her husband might not want to upset her by talking about the cancer every day because he loved her very much, she changed her statement as if she suddenly remembered. In fact he did tell her that the cancer was very advanced. She reached out for KKA's hand and holding it gently she stooped forward to create a posture of confession. She said that what she was going to tell had not been told to anyone. In fact she admitted that she never had the courage to mention it, because she was afraid of great embarrassment on her husband's behalf. She asked for my assurance that I would not tell anyone in case it might smear her husband's character. About 48 hours before her husband died, he was having a lot of pain. So the staff put him on a morphine pump. Later that evening she and her daughter noticed that the syringe was empty. At the same time the nurse came in and expressed her surprise. There should have been a lot more morphine left in that pump and she could not understand how it had emptied so early. The nurse dismissed the issue by saying that it could have happened by accident and filled it again. Mrs N and the daughter looked at each other and the daughter remarked to the nurse, whether the patient might have done it deliberately to overdose himself. The nurse made some gesture, which Mrs N took as that might be the case. Mrs N accounted the incident as her husband had done something criminal. When KKA assured her that such an accident was not uncommon in his experience, as electronic machines might sometime misbehave. She was happy to accept that and redeemed her husband from embarrassment.

Only after removing all minor issues the most important guilt became exposed. The dam of tears burst and she said, "I should not have gone home. I should not have listened to my daughter. I should have stayed. The hospital phone rang only an hour or so after I got home. I knew then that he had gone. By the time we got to the hospital he was peaceful." That guilt of leaving him to die alone, which in her judgement was an enormous and unpardonable neglect. KKA asked her to think hard and to tell every detail barring any judgement details. Then she vividly remembered that he was comfortable at the time she left the hospital and he had very clearly gestured to her that it was all right for her to go home. He was unable to say much as he was drifting in and out of consciousness. But she assumed that he was bidding goodbyes to her. Most importantly she remembered again that he had a smile on his face and he looked contented. In fact Mrs N with her daughter stayed with him in the hospital all day long and were exhausted. There was nothing more to be done. The daughter had to go home to see to her children. Judging from the gestures made by her husband it was all right for them to go home, as he was comfortable. So they went home. At that time everything seemed to be the right thing to do.

KKA introduced the usual argument in such a situation that one could only do whatever seemed to be the right thing to do at any precise moment in time. What people overlook that any living creature, including human beings could do only one act at one moment in time. Everyone without exception had to make that choice of "*only one decision*" and "*to carry out that decision*". Therefore it is totally unfair and wrong to create guilt and to pass the verdict of "you are guilty" on something, which was done with all the good intentions and the true belief of that it was the right thing to do at that precise moment. In the case of Mrs N, the guilty verdict could only be passed if she did that choosing solely because she did not love him and did not care about him before. It would be preposterous even to attempt to suggest that, a fact that she knew it well in her heart. Equally it would be preposterous to attempt to suggest that with all the love and care she carried in her heart, her decision to go home leaving her husband in a hospital bed, which she believed to be the most reasonable thing to do was wrong and culpable of neglect. KKA suggested that Mrs N needed to put things in their true perspective. Under no circumstance she could ever be guilty. KKA could make that statement only after giving the full explanations and arguments as described.

On the other hand, without spending much time on explanations and proper reasoning, many people would normally make comments like - "oh, don't be silly", "how would you know that he was going to die", "you shouldn't feel guilty" and so on. The bereaved would dismiss such comments straight away. They will not accept anything but they will stick with their verdict of guilty for the reasons, which KKA have discussed elsewhere. Mrs N had no hesitation to accept the explanations and rephrase her understanding that she had never thrown away her love towards him by leaving the hospital. The proof of that love was obvious by suffering from the extreme grief. Mrs N did not have any hesitation to throw away her guilt. She spontaneously appeared very relaxed and smiling. She let her shoulders down and said "what a relief, a great load on my mind has gone. Thank you."

At that stage she looked at ease. Further direct questioning clearly revealed that she had no further negative issues, except she wanted to say goodbye to her husband as a final act with him. KKA took Mrs N through the last stage of the Question and Answer Model of properly saying goodbye. She was much relieved and contented. She did not require any medication and in fact she felt so much better that she started with an active and happy life.

CASE NO 11

It is not uncommon that the bereaved may feel guilty after leaving the bedside for a short time the death occurs. After waiting for hours at the bedside of the patient and noticing nothing is happening indicative of death, they may think that it will be alright to leave the bedside for quite justifiable reasons. Looking back they would be kicking themselves because, if they had stayed for another hour or so they would not have missed the actual moment of their loved one passing away. It makes them feel unforgivably guilty and then will continue to suffer from harmful grief because of that self-imposed guilty verdict.

In the case of Mrs B she had spent all day with her elderly and seriously ill husband in the hospital. Late that evening her husband compelled her to go home for a little rest. While she was about to leave he called her back, kissed her and said, "Goodbye, take care of yourself". Mrs B was exhausted and did not take much notice of the way he said goodbye. Within an hour after she had reached home, the hospital telephoned her to let her know that her husband had passed away peacefully. She felt very guilty, as in her own words, that 'she had done the greatest injustice to their loving relationship of 60 years standing'. Mrs B's harmful grief presented as various physical illnesses, which did not respond to any form of treatment. During the grief therapy, KKA was able to remove her harmful grief. He explained to her that often the deceased would have a premonition of their impending death. According to common belief, when people die, they might show great struggle and the scene might be very upsetting for anyone to witness, especially by someone whom he much loved. It was not difficult for KKA to convince Mrs B that her husband loved her very much and he knew that she felt the same way. Because of that great love, he did not want her to remember how death came to him. Instead he wanted his sweetheart to have her last memory of him as saying goodbye and not of him unconscious and struggling to the end. He might have known that he was going to die very soon, which he deliberately wanted to hide from her. Mrs B was very happy not only to accept the explanation but also she believed it as the truth. Finally KKA helped her to say a proper goodbye, which was one important thing she had missed. Mrs B lived happily looking after her grandchildren for the rest of her life until she died peacefully at a ripe old age.

CASE NO 12
This case illustrates a very common presentation of guilt provoking a scenario of making decisions either against the wish of the deceased or to

the contrary of giving way to the wish of the deceased against the wish of the bereaved.

Mr A was eighty years of age, when KKA helped him with his harmful grief. Even though KKA had known Mr A for many years and that his wife, Mrs M had passed away five years prior to the treatment. His daughter had indicated to KKA that her father remained depressed and ever since the death of Mrs M he had not shown any interest in the many hobbies he used to have. He presented as tired all the time and easily got snappy with people. As an intelligent person, though Mr A was aware of what was going on in him, he was afraid to discuss the issue with anyone. What had come out from the treatment was that, he was almost disabled to talk about his feelings because of the terrible guilt that he was carrying in relation to Mrs M's death. He was very ashamed and felt that people would judge him as weak and unloving.

One day, he called to see KKA pretending that the visit was friendly and casual. But KKA picked up clues from his body language that he wanted to talk about his grief. Guessing correctly, KKA helped him to breakout from his fearful silence by directly asking him how he was coping with the loss of his wife? Mr A, through a cascade of tears, admitted that not a single minute passed by during the past five years without grieving and crying. On that day he needed to tell his "crime", but did not know how? He hoped KKA would do something!

Straight away KKA introduced the Question and Answer model in full. After talking about a few trivial issues, Mr A broke down with extreme shame and guilt because in his judgement he had done a great injustice to his wife. They had lived a blissful, happy and loving married life for over fifty years. When Mrs M became very ill with respiratory failure, she insisted that she stayed at home. She told him in confidence that her greatest wish was to die in her own home. Mr A and his daughter wanted her to get treated in hospital because they believed that she had more chance of being comfortable in the hospital. As extreme love dictated, Mrs M's unrelenting insistence as her last wish, Mr A took sides with her and kept her at home against the wish of the others. During the last few minutes leading to the death of Mrs M, she appeared to be distressed even though she was unconscious. After her death, drowned in extreme sadness, Mr A blamed himself for causing distress to Mrs M even though it only happened for a short period preceding her departure. He should have sent her to the hospital by ignoring the wish of Mrs M. Automatically the judgement of enormous guilt against the serious blame took residence in his thoughts and feeling day in and day out.

KKA quoted the Book in Heaven and the Boat metaphors. KKA was able to make Mr A understand and accept that there was no guarantee that she might have got any better comfort in the hospital, authenticated by the experience of KKA in the medical practice over many years. Moreover she could have died in the ambulance rattling along the long distance to the nearest hospital. Most probably Mr A might not be sitting in the ambulance and holding her hand during her last moments. Possibly she might have died in such strange surroundings and with strange people to attend to her. On one hand, all those things could be the worst thing for a dying person or on the other hand, her wish happened to be the best, as far as Mrs M was concerned, because her beloved Mr A was sitting next to her holding her hand and saying goodbye as she closed her eyes. Mr A did not take any more time to declare that he no longer needed to feel guilty of what he thought initially as the wrong act, which he did towards his wife. After all, knowing what he had done turned out to be the best for his wife, the relief from his guilt and hurt and the contentment of having fulfilling the last wish of his loved one was immeasurable.

After thanking KKA profusely, Mr A revealed that he had been searching for a way to get out of his terrible grieving for the past three years. He had read many books and visited a few libraries, but he could not find an answer to make him to feel normal. He could not believe, that KKA had achieved in one hour what he had searched for three years. Mr A also iterated that people can only perceive one side of everything, most of the time the wrong interpretation, when someone had to endure extreme hurt and pain from the demise of the loved one. KKA agreed and replied with a metaphor. *"It is impossible to have a dinner plate or a coin with only one side. But the pain will stop the people from wanting even to look for the other side of the plate, until some else like me exposed the possibility. A little explanation goes a long way"*.

In another case the son decided to send his father to the hospital against the wish of the father and mother. The father died on the way to hospital. The guilt was heavy and started the harming process by the son presenting with severe asthma. Until then he had not suffered from any illness to mention. When KKA treated the son in a similar manner as in case No.12, his asthma got such a lot better needing only occasional medication.

CASE NO. 13
This case presented as flight phobia.

Mrs S was known to KKA for a few years. During one of their family reunions everyone was talking about holidays. Her husband mentioned to KKA that they only could go away to places where they could drive to, because Mrs S had suffered from severe flight phobia. She was in her early seventies and in good health. Mrs S was eager to get over her fear and really wished to fly and to visit far away countries. She agreed to explore the reasons for her phobia.

During the analysis, she revealed that her fear was based on a deep feeling that she never wanted her young children to grow up without their mother. The flight phobia was not an issue for many years because family finances could not have accommodated such trips.

When her children were grown up and they became wealthy and able to afford far away holidays and only then she realised that she had a severe fear of flying. She did not have any insight into her phobia, which even prohibited her from asking for any form of therapeutic help until she spoke to KKA to whom she held in high regard. She already knew about his expertise in such matters.

Further analysis to find out the underlying dynamics of the feeling of orphaning her children she was reminded of her own childhood. Her mother died suddenly when she was only six years of age. Her father died within a year of her mother's death. She and her two brothers were split up to live with their aunties and uncles. To add to her sadness and fear, none of the adults who were in contact with her during her growing up period, ever talked about her parents especially anything connected with their deaths. Mrs S, with full of surprise, admitted that she had not had the slightest insight into the connection between her phobia and the loss of her own parents until the occasion when KKA had helped her. She also admitted that she always carried a kind of fear of the unknown as well as lacking in confidence. Almost straight away she expressed grief, which she still suffered. She wished that it would be wonderful if she could say goodbye to her mother. Mrs S was not allowed to see her mother after her death as she died in the hospital and the adults did not allow Mrs S to attend the funeral without any explanation. KKA offered her his package of grief treatment. She became a changed person and wished she had talked to KKA many years ago!

CASE NO. 14
This case is about the journey of grief in a child.

SK was only eight years of age when her father, MK, became unexpectedly ill. Unexpectedly, because he was big and strong and everyone who knew him believed that nothing could make him ill. Within two weeks of him being ill, he was diagnosed with untreatable cancer. He died in hospital in a matter six months. In that young age, SK was bewildered by not knowing what was going on, apart from all the family members looked sad and numb. All SK was able to understand was that her father was becoming very weak. She guessed that he was in a lot of pain but he was putting on a brave face especially in the presence of her. Towards the end of his life he spent a lot time in the hospital for specialised treatments.

Within a few months after the death of MK, SK received counselling therapy for a few months to help her to cope with the grief. She appeared to be all right for the next year or so, apart from occasional outbursts of crying or being angry over trivial incidents. Later on she found it unable to cope with schooling. Her performance fell to a very low level, failing badly in the schoolwork and overtly expressing emotional outbursts. At that stage of grief she was brought to the attention KKA for help.

The reoccurring questions troubling her tender mind were about the nature of cancer, especially related to the specific cancer, which caused the death of her father. She wanted to know what is cancer and how her father could get one? Whether the cancer was caused by exposure to chemicals associated with the job of MK? She was asking herself, whether the cancer and so the death of MK might have been prevented? KKA explained and answered all the questions in a language a child of her age would understand. She was satisfied with the explanations given by KKA. Then she wanted to know how did MK die, because she was not present at the time of the death. It also meant that SK missed saying goodbye to him. From the explanations and descriptions given by KKA, she was helped to realise that the death was inevitable, though getting the cancer was most unfortunate and nothing could have been done to prevent it. KKA helped her to say goodbye and reinforced her need to believe that how much MK did love her. SK started showing remarkable improvement in her school-work and showed greatly improved emotional stability.

For the following three or so years SK did well in coping with growing up into her early teenage years. SK was good in her sports, but contrary to her ability to excel in her performance, she lacked in confidence to progress with the higher technical part of the sport. On that occasion KKA was asked to help. Discussions revealed that she was still suffering from grief. The questions, which she was asking, were mainly about if anything more could have been done in his treatment, especially for pain relief during the last few days. She also wanted to clarify whether the hospital were competent. KKA had the benefit of knowing the details of the treatment and care, which MK had received. Her questions arose from hearsay and he was able to dispel her doubts and reassure her about the truth, which was MK, did receive the best he could have had. KKA trained SK in self-hypnosis to strengthen her faith in herself and believe in her own strength and ability. She chose certain memories of her father, especially how strong and good a person he was, for her to use as an anchor in self-hypnosis for improving her confidence. Once again, she showed great improvement not only in her sports but also in all aspects of her life.

SK remained very positive in her life and was able to continue with higher education. However, once again SK found herself feeling down and getting angry at trivial incidents, which she felt were not like her personality. She became miserable because she found herself unable to control her outbursts of anger. Her education also suffered. As she was approaching nineteen years of age and realising she needed to take positive steps for a future career, she asked for help from KKA. On analysis it was revealed that she has been suffering from grief due to a different issue yet to be resolved. More questions and reassurances on previous answers were asked for. Only after hearing those answers once again, it was revealed to her the unresolved issue, which was that she was missing her father. KKA pointed out to SK that all her life she would be carrying the vital genes from her father, and some genes would have imprints of her father's strength, wisdom and assertiveness, by which he could have

achieved anything he would have wanted. Thus the knowledge transmit-
ted through genes, which her father had given to her, would provide her
with all the guidance she needed to get what she wanted in her career
and all her life, as if her father were with her all the time. SK was very
contented with her fresh understanding and she was able to attain a very
successful career move at the age of nineteen.